AF838683

RHEUMATOLOGY

Educational Communications
P.O. Box 87
Pomona, New York 10970
(914) 354-7446

Problems in Primary Care Series

Other books in the series

Cardiology, Thomas H. Lee, Jr., MD, 1990.
ISBN: 0-87489-463-8

Neurology, James L. Bernat, MD and Frederick M. Vincent, MD, 1987.
ISBN: 0-87489-407-7

Otolaryngology, edited by D. Thomas Upchurch, MD. FACS, 1989.
ISBN: 0-87489-442-5

Pulmonary Medicine, edited by Robert D. Brandstetter, MD, 1989.
ISBN: 0-87489-468-9

Urology, edited by Elroy D. Kursh, MD and Martin I. Resnick, MD, 1987.
ISBN: 0-87489-419-0.

RHEUMATOLOGY

PROBLEMS IN PRIMARY CARE

MATTHEW H. LIANG, MD, MPH

W. NEAL ROBERTS, MD

CELESTE ROBB–NICHOLSON, MD, MPH

LORI BANNON, MD

MEDICAL ECONOMICS BOOKS
Oradell, New Jersey 07649

Library of Congress Cataloging-in-Publication Data
Rheumatology: problems in primary care/Matthew N. Liang ... [et al.].
p. cm.
ISBN 0-87489-421-2
1. Rheumatology—Handbooks, manuals, etc. 2. Musculoskeletal system—Diseases—Handbooks, manuals, etc. I. Liang, Matthew H.
[DNLM: 1. Arthritis. 2. Bone Diseases. 3. Rheumatism. WE 544 R4718]
RC925.R48 1989
616.7'23—dc20
DNLM/DLC
for Library of Congress 89-13076
CIP

ISBN 0-87489-421-2

Medical Economics Company Inc.
Oradell, New Jersey 07649

Printed in the United States of America

Copyright © 1990 by Medical Economics Company Inc., Oradell, N.J. 07649. All rights reserved. None of the content of this publication may be reproduced, stored in a retrieval system, or transmitted in any form or by any means (electronic, mechanical, photocopying, recording, or otherwise) without the prior written permission of the publisher.

The authors and publisher have exerted every effort to ensure that drug selection, dosage, and therapeutic modalities set forth in this text are in accord with current recommendations and practice at the time of publication. However, in view of ongoing research, changes in government regulations, and the constant flow of information relating to drug therapy, and drug reactions, the reader is urged to check the package insert for each drug for any change in indications and dosage and for added warnings and precautions. This is particularly important when the recommended agent is a new or infrequently employed drug.

Contents

About the Authors

Matthew H. Liang, MD, MPH is Associate Professor of Medicine at Harvard Medical School, Medical Director of Rehabilitation Services at the Brigham and Women's Hospital, Director of the Robert B. Brigham Multipurpose Arthritis Center, and Lecturer in the Department of Health Policy and Management at Harvard School of Public Health. He is a general internist and rheumatologist. His research interests include public health aspects of rheumatic disease disability, clinical epidemiology, and clinical decision making.

Neal Roberts, Jr., MD is an Assistant Professor of Medicine at the Medical College of Virginia and a full time member of the Division of Rheumatology. He is the 1988 winner of the Dubois Research Prize of the American College of Rheumatology and is an active clinical investigator in rheumatology.

Celeste R. Robb-Nicholson, MD, MPH is an Instructor of Medicine at Harvard Medical School, a general internist in the Department of Medicine at the Brigham and Women's Hospital and course director of the Musculoskeletal Pathophysiology Course for Harvard Medical School. She is doing research on fatigue in systemic rheumatic diseases.

Lori Bannon, MD was a fourth year Harvard Medical Student at the time this book was started and has now finished three years of anesthesiology training. Following completion of Fellowships in obstetrics and pediatric anesthesia at the Brigham and Women's Hospital and Boston Children's Hospital, she will be Chief Resident in Anesthesia at The Massachusetts General Hospital.

Foreword

A central responsibility of the primary care physician is to interpret the illness experience of the patient and make the correct translation into the disease classifications of medicine. What the patient interprets as an illness may have as much to do with dysfunctional relationships or unhappy life experiences as with pathology of biologic systems. Or, the patient may minimize some symptom that is the harbinger of a serious, even life-threatening, disorder while attributing the symptom to a troubled social situation. Nowhere are the skills of the clinician challenged more than in forming an accurate assessment of the true significance of an ache or pain in the musculoskeletal system. The authors of *Rheumatology: Problems in Primary Care* provide an excellent road map to assist the busy practitioner in making these assessments and in developing the appropriate management plan of patient education, treatment, or referral to a specialist.

Musculoskeletal problems are very common in primary care practice. Acute sprains and strains alone ranked ninth in frequency (2.4% of all ambulatory encounters) in the National Ambulatory Care Survey.[1] In the Virginia Study, 118 family physicians recorded all health care problems encountered in their practices during a two-year period.[2] The distribution of diagnostic categories was remarkably constant across rural, suburban, and urban practices. Of the 526,196 problems recorded, more than 34,000 were musculoskeletal or rheumatologic (6.46% of all encounters). Sprains and strains ranked sixth in frequency (12,830 cases) among the 567 discrete coding categories. Among the 75 most common medical problems were fibrositis, rheumatoid arthritis, osteoarthritis, "other arthritis," and back pain without radiation to the lower extremity. Each

---

[1] Rosenblatt RA, Cherkin DC, Schneeweiss R, Hart LG. The content of ambulatory care in the United States: an interspecialty comparison. N Engl J Med 1983; 309:892–97.

[2] Marsland DW, Wood M, and Mayo F. A data bank for patient care, curriculum, and research in family practice: 526,196 patient problems. J Family Practice 1976; 3:25–37.

patient complaint presented as a diagnostic problem for the physician who then had to decide to treat and manage the problem or refer the patient to a subspecialist.

In time each primary care physician defines the boundary of clinical problems for his or her practice. The intellectual interests of the physician, the ready availability of subspecialists in rheumatology or orthopedics, and the degree of confidence in the requisite skills and knowledge to diagnose and manage a given problem shape the boundaries for each of us. This text, with its emphasis on the presenting symptoms rather than the pathophysiology, will make the domain of rheumatologic disease more accessible to the primary care physician. The easier access will undoubtedly spark intellectual curiosity to learn more about the broad array of musculoskeletal problems that present so commonly in community practice. Most importantly, the clinician who uses this text will become more confident in managing these problems and more precise in defining the point at which the patient should be referred. The outcome should be better informed patients, more appropriate treatment, and greater professional satisfaction.

Robert S. Lawrence, M.D.
Charles S. Davidson Associate Professor of Medicine
Harvard Medical School
Director, Division of Primary Care, Harvard Medical School
Chief of Medicine, The Cambridge Hospital

Preface

This is a book about the management of the most common musculoskeletal complaints and conditions in ambulatory medicine. A physician of first contact, whether a pediatrician, family practitioner, internist, obstetrician, or subspecialist, needs to manage these problems efficiently and effectively. The natural history of many common complaints suggests that the majority have a benign outcome. This does not mean they are self-limited or trivial. For the patient, common conditions are trivial only in retrospect, after they have been evaluated and treated competently. Seemingly benign complaints inappropriately managed may lead to physical or emotional morbidity, or even death. A trivial complaint may be the early symptom of a life-threatening illness or a proxy for emotional problems. Management strategies that do not take into account the probabilities of a rare but *treatable* condition may jeopardize a patient's health.

A trivial illness is an important experience that, if not successfully coped with by the patient, may set up a pattern of sickness behavior and/or dependency. If every symptom is made into a "disease" by an inappropriate diagnostic label, the patient is more likely to view common symptoms as serious illnesses. If every symptom is treated with medication, the patient is likely to expect a pill for every ill. If the physician says, "You came just in time" or "You should have come sooner," the individual is likely to doubt his or her own common sense and to become dependent. An illness is an opportunity for the physician to teach and for the patient to learn, as well as an opportunity to increase that patient's competence in self-care.

The generalist is accessible to his or her patients and assumes responsibility for all aspects of their health care. The generalist must know the boundaries of his or her competence and refer when appropriate. The physician in an ambulatory setting makes the crucial determination as to whether a constellation of symptoms and signs is a "disease" or not. In this role, the physician is frequently confronted with vague symptoms and nonspecific signs, which must be evaluated to make an operational decision within the time of an office visit.

Many rheumatological conditions defy simple diagnosis and most defy precise confirmation. Uncertainty characterizes the usual conditions under which decisions are made in an ambulatory setting. Intimate knowledge of a patient and the ability to follow up the patient enable the generalist to make management decisions that a consultant seeing patient for a single episode would never entertain.

The specific content of what the generalist does will depend on what conditions are prevalent in the community and what a generalist has to treat because of the unavailability of specialty care.

Physicians are often too dependent on technology and procedures. They overevaluate without regard to the consequences of discovering asymptomatic conditions; medicate without knowledge of nondrug modalities; overmanage patients and make them too dependent; and dwell upon the process rather than the outcome of their intervention, and upon the disease rather than its functional consequences.

Studies in the ambulatory setting in different countries show remarkably similar patterns of morbidity. The organization of this book is based on the U.S. National Ambulatory Medical Care Survey and encompasses about 80% of the presenting musculoskeletal complaints to office-based physicians.

For each symptom or problem, the central questions for *the initial visit* to the office are, What is the *most likely* diagnosis? and What treatable conditions can I *not* afford to miss?

Treatable conditions and clues to their diagnosis are highlighted by tables of Red Flags or Don't Miss conditions. Experience in the practice of rheumatology and general internal medicine has led us to also suggest referral criteria to identify situations in which a more experienced specialist should be consulted or should assume the primary responsibility for care. Understanding one's limitations is essential for both the generalist and the specialist. Explicitly coordinated care in which the primary doctor and the consultant understand their responsibilities can be a rich learning experience for both and is ultimately the best for the patient.

The joint examination, usually glossed over in medical school and housestaff programs, is the key to diagnosis and management of rheumatic complaints. It is our experience that this skill is best learned from a skilled examiner, and a picture or diagram cannot communicate this fully. Short of a practicum, however, the reader is referred to Stanley Hoppenfeld's *Physical Examination of the Spine and Extremities*, Appleton-Century-Crofts, New York 1976, an excellent practical book with pictures that teach.

Finally, this text is intended to complement the vast number of excellent textbooks of rheumatology and orthopedics that discuss primarily diseases rather than symptoms. We felt little need to duplicate these texts. Rather, ours is a practical road map oriented to community-based, nonreferral practice.

Our special thanks to Mary Scamman and Jacqueline Pepe Mazzie who deserve a bouquet for each "final" revision that they cheerfully completed.

ONE

Musculoskeletal complaints

1

Sorting Out Musculoskeletal Complaints

One out of every seven visits to the primary care physician is for musculoskeletal pain. Of these, the vast majority are nonarticular rheumatic syndromes, such as bursitis, tendinitis, fibrositis, or low back and neck pain. Inflammatory arthritis and connective tissue diseases are infrequent. Consequently, the goals of sorting out these complaints are to rule out treatable illnesses, to identify which patients need more extensive diagnostic tests and follow-up, and to treat to prevent dysfunction.

To do this, x-rays and laboratory tests are rarely of help and are often impractical in a busy office. The key to sorting out musculoskeletal complaints is a careful history, particularly regarding precipitating factors, the specific areas that hurt; what makes the pain worse or better; the temporal sequence of symptoms (Figure 1–1); and the exclusion of systemic illness. Laboratory tests are almost never indicated on the initial visit and x-rays are only important in certain situations (Table 1–1). The second most useful part of the clinical evaluation is a joint examination to identify the anatomic structure(s) involved and to identify inflammatory synovitis, joint instability, and localized tenderness.

This text is organized by the major presenting symptom patterns and gives an approach to identifying treatable illnesses. For each symptom, the most common causes in an unselected, community-based practice are listed. A series of red flags based on unusual history, symptoms, or physical findings should alert the physician to illnesses that require early recognition and treatment. Finally, a plan for treatment that emphasizes physical and medical management, the prevention of functional disability, patient education goals, and referral criteria follows.

HISTORY

The goals of the history are to find clues to whether the pain is inflammatory or noninflammatory, how and when the pain started, what makes the pain worse or

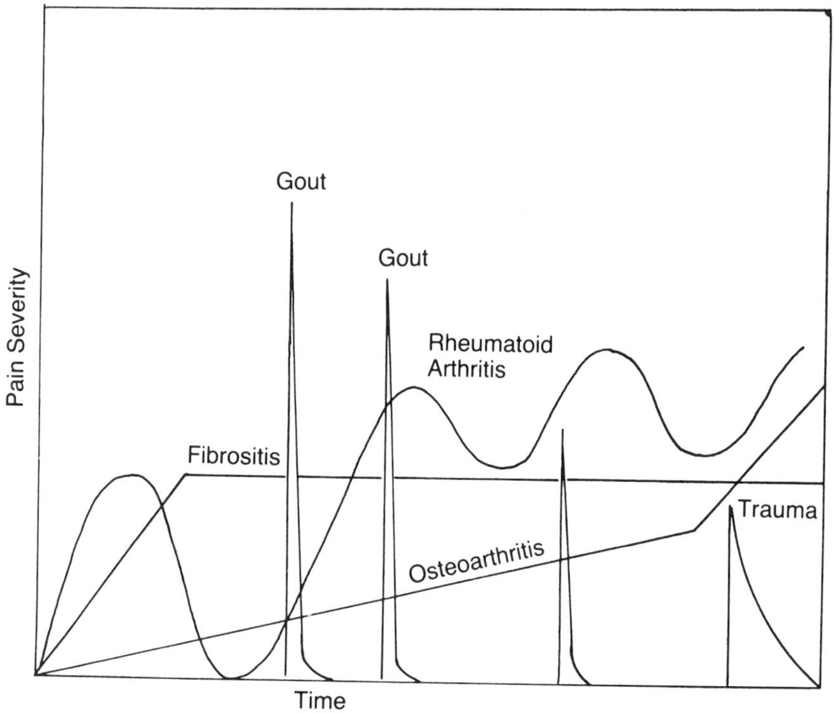

Figure 1–1. Variability over time is characteristic of diseases such as rheumatoid arthritis or bursitis and is distinguished from the more constant time course of osteoarthritis. Osteoarthritis may worsen dramatically toward the end of the course, but the pain never remits for any prolonged period. Fibrositis is even more constant, whereas gout produces a distinctive spiking course over time.

better, its temporal pattern, and the presence of systemic symptoms such as fever or weight loss, which would suggest that the arthritis is part of a systemic illness.

Identify the location of the pain by having the patient point to what hurts. People may not be able to distinguish pain from a joint or from other structures without help. If the patient can identify a discrete area, that is helpful and should be confirmed by physical examination.

Arthralgia implies pain originating from or around the joint but not necessarily that the pain comes from within the joint itself. Pain originating from joint structures should be improved by resting the joint and made worse by stretching the joint or by weight bearing. Stiffness after prolonged immobility ("gelling") suggests inflammatory joint disease or synovitis. This symptom probably results from altered viscosity of inflammatory joint fluid, but is also described in older patients and in patients with hypothyroidism, Parkinson's disease, and disorders

TABLE 1–1. INDICATIONS FOR RADIOGRAPHIC EVALUATION OF MUSCULOSKELETAL COMPLAINTS

Severe trauma
Age < 15 or > 45 at onset
No focal findings around joint structures
Symptoms not relieved by rest of involved area
Prepubertal patient

with only a minor inflammatory component such as osteoarthritis. Clinically significant gelling lasts more than 15 to 30 minutes. Patients with florid synovitis can describe both little or no gelling or gelling that lasts all day. In inflammatory disease the length of gelling may be proportional to the severity of the inflammatory process and may shorten as the patient improves. When asking about morning stiffness, ask the patient for the usual time of awakening, then the time that the patient is as limber as he or she will be during the day. The time between these two points is the amount of morning stiffness and is more reliable than a casual question such as, "How much stiffness do you have," or "How long does your stiffness last?"

Night pain is a cardinal symptom because it usually leads to a discrete and treatable diagnosis. Pain that awakens the patient can be neurogenic, vascular, infectious, or crystalline disease (gout, pseudogout) or can be due to severe structural joint damage. Tendonitis and bursitis can also awaken a patient. Synovitis without structural damage rarely wakes a patient. Neurogenic pain is described in vague terms ("I can't describe it.") or as numbness, extremity falling asleep, shooting pain, or pins and needles, etc. Pain that comes from vascular insufficiency of whatever cause is brought on by use and is relieved with rest within a couple of seconds. Symptoms caused by peripheral vascular disease may sound like those of spinal stenosis, but, in the latter, use-related pain is usually bilateral, usually does not radiate below the knee, and rest improves the symptoms slowly.

"Giving Way or Locking"

A complaint of "giving way" at the knee or hip needs to be distinguished between giving way *without warning*, which occurs with an unstable knee or muscle weakness, versus giving way *with* pain, which may occur with meniscus tears and loose bodies within the joint.

Locking is the inability to take a joint smoothly through its complete range of motion because of an internal derangement (loose body, torn cartilage, or meniscus) or an extraarticular soft-tissue block such as a tendon nodule seen in trigger finger.

Weakness

At least three types of weakness are described by patients. The first is generalized weakness and easy fatigability, as may occur with disuse atrophy or the general deconditioning that occurs after systemic illness or myasthenia. The second is painless loss of power in a specific muscle group, as occurs in complete denervation and nerve-root damage (polio). The third type of weakness accompanies numbness or other neurological symptoms and implies a neuropathy such as in carpal tunnel and sciatica.

Weakness, Cramping, Aching

Cramping, spasms, muscle pain, aching, or myalgias may be equivalent depending on the patient's vocabulary and may not be distinguishable by the history alone. Cramping is a commonly experienced symptom. The most common is nocturnal cramps, an acute spasm and intense pain of the calf or intrinsic foot muscles relieved by stretching the muscle, time, heat, or massage. Spasm or cramping of the musculature crossing a joint forces the joint into flexion. Cramping of the intrinsic muscles of the feet forces the toes into plantar flexion. Spasm of paraspinous muscles of the low back causes secondary scoliosis. Cramping is acute and once the muscle is relaxed, it is over. On the other hand, muscle pain, myalgias, and aching are less intense, usually do not awaken the patient from sleep or prevent function, and are not use-related. Common examples of myalgias include those seen with bacterial or viral sepsis and the achiness that occurs after prolonged exertion. Cramping in an extremity muscle is almost always benign and self-limited. Cramping of multiple muscles, muscles of the abdomen, or muscles of the upper extremity implies a primary muscle disease or metabolic-toxic myopathy. Regional cramping and muscle pain may also be caused by arterial insufficiency, and a clue is its use-related nature.

Weakness, malaise, and tiredness are nonspecific symptoms and are frequently used interchangeably. Weakness implies a loss of power or endurance. The sufferer has difficulty initiating and maintaining a functional activity that requires strength. When a patient has weakness or decreased endurance of one extremity, he or she may have a neurological lesion, local muscle atrophy; or a disrupted musculoskeletal unit, such as a torn tendon or torn muscle (v13., rotator-cuff tear).

Some patients mention "weakness" when they mean decreased stamina or easy fatiguability. With regard to evaluating a potential muscle problem, these descriptions may be equivalent in significance, but they are also nonspecific symptoms of chronic diseases, probably related to deconditioning, toxic metabolic effects (uremia, anemia), or generalized myopathies, such as myasthenia gravis or a variety of muscle enzyme disorders characterized by deficiencies in anerobic glycolysis.

Weakness is frequently a term used by the patient for malaise, asthenia, or a

TABLE 1–2. FUNCTIONAL ASSESSMENT

How does your condition affect you?
Which activity is most difficult for you?
Are you worse, better, or the same as before?
What can't you do now that you could do before?
What can't you do, but need to or want to do?

nonspecific loss of well-being. A wide differential must be engaged if the physical exam shows no objective weakness.

Review of Systems

A brief screening review of systems is done to see whether the musculoskeletal symptom might be related to a systemic illness and also whether the area is the only joint involved. This can be done simply by asking:

- If you didn't have this (joint complaint) would you be feeling OK? or
- Is there anything else that is making you feel bad?
- Do you have any other medical problems that I should know about?
- Are there any other joints involved?

Functional Assessment (Table 1–2)

The evaluation is not over until one assesses how the symptoms affect the person's functioning in work, play, and home activities. Dysfunction is the final common pathway resulting from all forms of untreated arthritis and musculoskeletal conditions and, along with pain, of most concern to the patient. Identifying difficulty in this area may point the physician toward different or more aggressive treatment. In the patient with polyarthritis, a joint that is symptomatically out of proportion to the others may indicate advanced structural damage or possibly even an infection. Simple questions to screen for functional problems are listed in Table 1–2. For patients with cognitive difficulties or multiple disabilities or in the elderly, observation of essential activities may point to specific difficulties.

PHYSICAL EXAMINATION

The history, the physical examination, and time are the three most important and useful tests in the diagnosis and management of musculoskeletal disorders. Each chapter in this book outlines an incisive physical examination for specific problems, but basic principles are emphasized here. The point of the examination is to reproduce the pain in order to locate the anatomical site; to identify whether the symptoms come from inside the joint or from an extraarticular source; and to determine whether it is inflammatory or noninflammatory. The cardinal signs of an intraarticular process (synovitis) are an effusion (fluid), warmth, palpable swelling over the joint line, a diminished range of motion in all directions of the joint, and pain or swelling over all palpable areas of the joint capsule.

Point tenderness over anatomical sites of bursa is bursitis or a tear in a muscle or tendon. Tendinitis , on the other hand, is suggested by linear swelling, warmth, crepitus, a rub, and tenderness over the course of the tendon. Stretching the tendon should reproduce the pain. Muscle pain is diffuse and is not well localized by either the patient or the examiner. Weakness, if present (and it frequently is not), is a supporting symptom and suggests muscle or nerve involvement.

The difference between the active and passive range of motion has clinical significance. In a brief screening exam, the patient is asked to imitate the examiner as he or she takes the major joints through an active range of motion. If there is no limitation or pain (look at the face), the joint need not be examined, except to look for subtle signs of inflammation when the suspicion is high. If the active range of motion is limited, one should note whether it is limited by pain, weakness, or mechanical block. The patient should then be taken through a passive range of motion. If the passive range is normal and the active range is limited, suspect a muscle or neurological problem, i.e., myopathy, torn ligament and muscle, or peripheral neuropathy. If the active range equals the passive range, suspect a soft-tissue mechanical block such as in a frozen shoulder or synovitis.

Another useful examination is to appreciate the "end feel" at the extreme of the range of motion. The distinction is made between a "hard" end feel versus a "soft" end feel. The hard end feel is abrupt, firm, and suggests a structural block such as osteoarthritis. More effort by the examiner to overcome the block fails and may result in pain. A soft end feel, in contrast, is the feel of an automobile clutch, in that the range is limited but can be overcome with slow force. The soft end feel is the typical feel of synovitis without significant structural damage.

The problem of differentiating between edema, cellulitis, and synovitis comes up frequently. Synovitis has signs of inflammation (dolor, calor, rubor, tumor) over the visible, palpable areas of the joint capsule. The swelling does not usually extend beyond the confines of the anatomical joint space except when tendon sheaths are involved. Rubor, a sign of classic inflammation, is not common in synovitis, except in crystalline synovitis or joint infection. Cellulitis, in contrast, has diffuse red swelling with or without a margin between the normal and the inflamed skin, occasionally with lymphangitis, and with regional lymphadenopathy. Pinching the skin gently away from the joint margin may cause discomfort. Edema, on the other hand, is bland swelling that goes beyond the confines of the joint margin and is frequently associated with pitting without redness or local warmth. The three — edema, cellulitis, and synovitis — may coexist in a given patient, and synovitis may need to be confirmed by aspirating the joint. One would not do this without prior antibiotic coverage if there is any question of overlying cellulitis. There is usually an area of the joint space that can be entered without passing through potentially infected skin. Consultation is wise.

TABLE 1–3. DIFFERENTIAL DIAGNOSIS OF MONOARTHRITIS

Traumatic

Fracture
Internal derangement
Tendonitis/bursitis
Hemarthrosis

Inflammatory

Infection — bacterial, viral, fungal, Lyme
Inflammatory arthritis
  crystalline (gout, pseudogout, etc.)
  RA/JRA
  SLE
  pallindromic
  etc.

Bone/Cartilage

Osteoarthritis
Avascular necrosis
Loose bodies
Tumor

Monoarthritis

A patient who complains of pain, stiffness, or a single swollen joint presents a broad differential that includes extraarticular conditons such as overuse syndromes and arthritis such as monarticular rheumatoid arthritis or Reiter's syndrome. The differential diagnosis in approximate order of frequency in a primary care setting is given in Table 1–3.

The patient's age is key in interpretation of the history. A young sexually active person may have gonococcal arthritis. Monoarticular complaints in prepubertal patients require careful evaluation for traumatic conditons and congenital defects such as a slipped capital epiphysis and hip dysplasia. The patient's age orders the probabilities of the differential and helps rule out specific diseases. One rarely thinks of crystal-induced arthridites, intermittent hydroarthritis, and gonococcal arthritis in prepubertal patients, for example. Sex, like age, is useful for ordering diagnostic possibilities within the differential diagnostic list, but is not strong enough to rule out certain conditions. Gout or Reiter's syndrome is less common in females, for example, but it occurs. Race and socioeconomic status are not strongly associated with particular arthridites and are much less useful than age and sex.

The degree of pain and the circumstances with which it occurs are very helpful clues to diagnoses. Severe pain and/or severe pain at rest narrows the differential but implies infection, until proven otherwise, or possibly crystal-induced synovitis (gout and pseudogout). Mild-to-moderate pain is seen in inflammatory monoarthridites and also in many other causes, such as hemarthrosis, tendonitis, and ligamentous strains.

The duration of the complaint may be helpful, as pain that has been present for weeks is not gout, but could be tophaceous gout (Figure 1–1) or is unlikely to be bacterial infectious arthritis, but could be tuberculosis or fungal arthritis.

A patient with complaints of arthritis may, in fact, have *poly*arthritis by history or examination. Do not miss this, as it may be a clue to a systemic arthritis. The physical examination is the single most important clinical tool to assess whether the symptom is inflammatory or noninflammatory, and if there is a moderate or larger effusion, it must be aspirated. Monoarthritis is an infection until proven otherwise. Only arthrocentesis for culture can definitively rule out infection.

A single episode of bleeding in the joint should clear within several days to 1 week. Persistent blood after this point implies rebleeding and a coagulopathy needs to be considered.

Acute monoarthritis with fever is always an infection until proven otherwise. Gout may have associated fever but the temperature should not be greater than 101°F. In any case, a joint aspiration is a must for any patient with fever and monarthritis.

The workup of acute monoarthritis, even without fever, usually requires aspiration of the joint. There are exceptions but when there is any doubt joint aspiration is simple and diagnostic. The exceptions include *reliable* patients with little-to-moderate pain who have few signs or symptoms of inflammation, i.e., small effusions that are not warm; patients for whom the pain is not severe and is related primarily to the use of the joint rather than pain with rest; and the absence of constitutional symptoms such as rash or fever.

In classic podagra (inflammation of the first metatarsophalangeal joint), many clinicians might opt to treat the patient for gout and to follow them closely, i.e., over the next 48, since the incidence of infection in this joint is low. For example, arthrocentesis may be omitted in a reliable patient with previous podagra, with known risk factors (hyperuricemia, recent debauchery, surgery within the last week, dehydration, acidosis), where the involvement is clearly located to the first metatarsophalangeal joint and does not extend outside of the joint, where there are no skin breaks, where the temperature is not greater than 101°F, and where there has been no history of trauma.

Atypical features necessitating joint aspiration of the first metatarsophalangeal joint would include age less than 40, systemic symptoms, temperature greater than 101°F, evidence for a primary source of infection or local breakdown of skin; joint previously damaged with inflammatory arthritis; diabetes; prior surgery of the joint; and immunosuppressive therapy.

Technique of joint aspiration

Some general principles and tips should be kept in mind: The size of the needle depends on the size of the joint (25 gauge for small joints; 22 gauge for moderate-to large joints). When joint fluid is aspirated, a 22-gauge needle may suffice, but a chronic effusion that is likely to have viscous material is difficult to aspirate with needles less than 18 gauge.

The joint should be placed in the position that accommodates the largest volume of fluid. Wrist, metacarpal, interphalangeal and knee joints should be in slight flexion; other joints should be in a neutral position. Enter the joint to avoid the neurovascular bundle, tendons, and ligaments. Injecting medication into a tendon may delay healing and cause tendon rupture. If you cannot identify the tendon with confidence, do not attempt injection.

Although the procedure is sterile, only one glove needs to be kept sterile to palpate the landmarks, and this is necessary only if the anatomy is not well appreciated, such as in a chubby knee. Prior to cleansing the area, press the needle cover (which usually has an indentation) or a ballpoint pen with the writing tip retracted firmly to mark the spot to be aspirated. This impression will mark the target and will not be washed away by the sterile preparation. Standard preparation includes betadine followed by alcohol to dryness.

Local xylocaine anesthesia is almost never needed unless the patient is apprehensive or is a child, or a large-bore needle is used, or biopsy or irrigation is contemplated. It is more uncomfortable to anesthetize the area than it is to make an injection. Another way to make the injection as tolerable as possible is to wait for the alcohol to dry, stretch the skin firmly, and make the needle entry perpendiculr to the surface of the skin. To anesthesitize skin, an intradermal wheel with xylocaine 1% without epinephrine, ethyl chloride spray, or ice may be used. Do not neglect the value of distraction during the procedure; talk to the patient.

What to Do With the Joint Fluid (Table 1–4)

How joint fluids are processed, what "standard" tests are done, and the quality of joint fluid analysis are variable. If the joint fluid is important enough to get and the patient is put through the inconvenience, one should examine the fluid properly.

Whether the fluid is inflammatory or noninflammatory can be judged by the clinical picture and the physical properties of the fluid (Table 1–5). The joint has clinical signs of inflammation. Normal joint fluid has the consistency and color of egg white, and newspaper print can be read easily through the syringe or through a vial, whereas inflammatory fluids make it difficult or impossible to read through it. The string sign is elicited after the syringe has been withdrawn by pressing slowly on the plunger with the syringe needle held parallel to the floor until a drop appears at the end of the needle and falls. Normally the fluid should string for about two to three inches. The more inflammatory the fluid, the more waterlike the consistency, and the fluid will drip. The string sign can also be elicited by placing synovial fluid between the index finger and the thumb and pulling the fingers apart slowly. The mucin clot test is also a test of joint fluid viscosity and requires chemical reagents; it is rarely done anymore. Inspecting the fluid for cells and crystals can be done quickly by touching a heparinized microhematocrit tube to the fluid, blowing it out gently on a glass slip, and covering the drop with a cover slip. Cell counts greater than 40 per high-powered field suggests inflammation.

TABLE 1–4. SYNOVIAL FLUID EVALUATION

1. Collect as much synovial fluid as possible. Place some fluid in a tube with heparin and some in a plain, sterile tube
2. Culture synovial fluid
3. Gram stain centrifuged pellet for inspection
4. Wet preparation
   a. Scan with ordinary light microscopy
   b. Look for crystals with polarizing microscope
5. Leukocyte count and differential

TABLE 1–5. JOINT FLUID ANALYSIS RAPID OFFICE EXAMINATION

	Noninflammatory	Inflammatory
Joint examination	Tumor	Dolor Tumor Calor Rubor
Gross appearance	Can read print through joint fluid	Print blurred or obliterated
String test	Strings 1″ to 2″	Drips like water from syringe
Heparinized microhematocrit tube of unspun joint fluid	$<$ 40 WBC/hpf ($<$ 4000/cmm)	$>$ 40 WBC/hpf ($>$ 4000/cmm)

If a fluid is inflammatory, the minimum tests should be a formal cell count, a careful look for crystals (gout, pseudogout), and, almost always, culture.

To avoid contaminated cultures, process the fluid meticulously. As soon as the needle is removed from the site, the needle should be replaced with a sterile one. Any sterile container can be used if it is sent promptly to the laboratory. The only exception is suspected gonorrhea, in which case a Thayer–Martin culture plate can be planted with fresh material and put under CO_2 STAT. If only a minimal amount of fluid is obtained, place a sterile needle on the hub and send the entire syringe for culture.

In looking for crystals, search the slide carefully and for at least 5 minutes if crystalline disease is suspected. Crystals may be seen without a special microscope or polarization. To do this, cut the light down to exaggerate refractile materials by closing the diaphragm and lowering the condenser. In most gout, pine-needle-shaped crystals inside and outside of the white blood cells will be seen; pseudogout will appear as pleomorphic rhomboid crystals. Pieces of polarizing plastic can be put over the light source and the eyepiece of a conventional microscope for very little cost. (see also page 93.)

Send fluid for culture, cell count, crystal analysis, and gram stain. Sugar and protein are of little use for making decisions. However, if only a few drops can be obtained from a joint, squirt a small amount onto a slide for examination and send the remainder for culture. Once the fluid has been examined, it can be dried and gram stained. When crystalline disease is suspected and the tap is "dry," there may be a small amount of ooze from the puncture site; it is worthwhile to touch a glass slide to this material for microscopy, since crystals may be seen.

X-Rays

In contrast to arthrocentesis, radiographs for a new joint complaint are rarely helpful and should be done selectively (Table 1–1). Plain radiographs show changes in the bone and changes in the soft tissue less well. The soft-tissue changes confirm the physical exam. The changes in bone are erosions (such as occurs in rheumatoid arthritis), fractures, and primary and secondary bone tumors. It takes 6 months of inflammation to see erosions from inflammatory synovitis. An x-ray taken before this is rarely helpful. One exception is the patient who has had recurrent attacks of arthritis in a joint. A radiograph may demonstrate erosions typical of gout. X-rays in septic joints become abnormal 10 days to 2 weeks into the course, by which time all septic joints should have been diagnosed.

Other Diagnostic Tests

Except for synovial fluid analysis in some disorders, there is no laboratory test that is absolutely diagnostic of rheumatic disorders. A serum uric acid will not diagnose gout and never rules out the possibility of infection. Twenty percent of patients with acute gout have normal serum uric acid. A normal white blood cell count does not rule out an infectious arthritis. In patients with early rheumatoid arthritis presenting as monoarthritis, the rheumatoid factor may be negative, and many other conditions and normal patients may have a positive rheumatoid factor.

Polyarthritis

Polyarthritis is the involvement of three or more joints with synovitis and is distinct from polyarthralgias in which there are multiple joint complaints with no obvious inflammation. Acute polyarthritis is a diagnostic dilemma as it includes almost every disease of importance in rheumatology and many that are potentially life threatening and are associated with high morbidity. Acute arthritis of less than 6 weeks cannot be diagnosed with any certainty but can be benign, such as postviral arthritis. A complete history, physical, and diagnositc evaluation is always necessary if constitutional symptoms or symptoms referred to other organ systems exist.

The elements of the history that are particularly helpful in sorting out this presentation are the pattern of joint involvement, the temporal sequence, the course, the presence or absence of extraarticular symptoms or signs, and the functional consequences of the articular involvement.

The sequence of symptoms have three major patterns; additive, migratory, and intermittent. In additive arthritis, one obtains a history that new joints are added to previously involved joints. In migratory arthritis, it is implied that joints become symptomatic then subside and new ones appear. In intermittent arthritis, the symptoms come and go, and when they go there are virtually no signs or symptoms suggesting joint involement.

The patterns may coexist in the same patient, but when they dominate the clinical presentation they may suggest a specific diagnosis. For instance, an additive pattern is seen in patients with rheumatoid arthritis and systemic lupus and Still's disease; migratory arthralgias and arthritis is typical of patients with gonococcal sepsis and acute rheumatic fever, and is associated with bacterial endocarditis. Intermittent arthritis is typically seen in gout before it becomes tophaceous gout, in pseudogout, and in Mediterranean fever.

Which joints are involved and whether this joint pattern is symmetrical or nonsymmetrical over time can help limit the diagnostic possibilities. For instance, rheumatoid arthritis would be the most likely diagnosis in the patient with synovitis of the small joints of the hands, wrists (excluding the distal interphalangeal joints), elbow, knee, ankle, and feet. Distal interphalangeal joint involvement with only nobby joints but without synovitis is osteoarthritis. Asymmetric synovitis of knees and ankles with backache suggests spondlyarthropathies. Pattern recognition in polyarthritis is helpful but is not diagnostic, since there is overlap.

The patient with polyarthritis requires a full history and physical examination. The pace of diagnosis and management depends on whether other organs are involved, and thus a patient cannot be discharged until that data base is established. The detailed review of systems looks for other organ involvement and establishes that arthritis is part of a systemic disease. In multisystem disease, heart, lung, kidney, and brain involvement is usually more important than the management of the joint symptoms.

Once the other organ systems have been evaluated and the decision has been made how acutely ill the patient is, the final task for the practitioner is to assess the impact of the arthritis on the patient's ability to care for himself or herself, and to play, work, and do child care.

The usefulness of laboratory tests and x-rays is primarily for the patient who has had a long illness, who looks sick, or who has other system involvement. For these patients, systemic lupus or vasculitis are possible and one should not sleep until the results of simple laboratory tests have come back. The tests ordered are dictated by signs or symptoms, but some organs are relatively quiet and require laboratory evaluation (lung, kidney, hematologic, heart, liver). A complete blood count, erythrocyte sedimentation rate, tests of renal function and liver function, urinalysis, electrocardiogram, and chest x-ray is the minimum evaluation, and other testing should be dictated by clinical suspicion. If there is a temperature, cultures should be obtained.

Polyarthralgias

Polyarthralgia is a common but nonspecific symptom. The majority of these complaints have a biological explanation, and if one takes a good history and tries to identify the anatomical source, a good operational diagnosis is possible. Patients may report multiple joint symptoms as being related, whereas in fact they are regional musculoskeletal syndromes. Others present with polyarthralgias and forget that they have had polyarthritis or polyarthralgias in the past. Polyarthralgia/polymyalgia has an extensive differential diagnosis.

If the examination reveals signs of inflammation or synovitis, the approach outlined in Poly*arthritis* should be followed. If the symptoms are articular and cannot be located to bursa or tendon, then polyarthralgias exist.

With a duration of symptoms under 6 weeks, benign conditions such as postviral syndromes and postexertional syndromes are common. These benign syndromes are suggested in older patients and in those with constitutional symptoms or symptoms referable to other organ systems. Patients with greater than 6 weeks of symptoms and who continue to have a completely normal examination need a more complete evaluation.

Patients with no functional impairment nor objective findings on examination or with laboratory evaluation have benign arthralgias. The cause of these disorders may eventually be better understood, but one should not medicalize the condition unnecessarily. These patients do better with massage, heat, relaxation therapy, stretching, or aerobic conditioning programs and the like, than with medications. Some patients have fears of crippling illness or having a serious unrecognized disease. In these cases, it is best to address their concerns directly.

MUSCULOSKELETAL COMPLAINTS IN YOUNG PATIENTS

Although this book does not cover pediatrics, a primary care physician will see adolescents and young adults with musculoskeletal complaints. Spontaneous complaints of joint or musculoskeletal problems in young patients is unusual. When present, these complaints are usually due to trauma. The history that is so helpful in sorting out complaints in adults is less helpful in young patients. A variety of important diagnoses that can lead to disability and pain occur with greater frequency in youth. These diagnoses include congenital problems, osteochondritis, primary bone tumors, growth disturbances, and spontaneous infectious arthritis. Chronic inflammatory arthritis, such as juvenile rheumatoid arthritis and its subsets, may present in a variety of ways. The finding of inflammation in a joint requires special diagnosis and management beyond the experience of both primary care physicians and many rheumatologists.

Approach

Although the history may not always be reliable, inquire about symptoms of inflammatory disease. These would be symptoms that worsen with prolonged inactivity and that are improved by joint use. Other clues to inflammatory arthritis are symptoms that vary from day to day and from hour to hour, and ones that response to antiinflammatory agents. Although it is not universally true, complaints are usually minimized or attributed to trivial causes.

Mothers talk about "growing pains," but the physician must try to make a diagnosis before attributing complaints to growing pains.

When the symptoms and/or signs are confusing or conflicting, one should ask about the functional consequences of the symptoms or how the family reacts when the youth complains. Signs or symptoms that do not make sense may be a sign of school or family stress, sometimes learned behavior from parents or siblings. Symptoms may be used by the child to get attention or affection.

On physical examination, if the patient has constitutional symptoms or looks sick, a full physical examination is required. If there are no constitutional symptoms, a complete joint exam should be performed. In someone with monoarticular complaints, do not miss referred pain. If one can find clear evidence of a soft-tissue lesion, tendinitis, bursitis, or localized muscle tenderness, further evaluation is usually not needed. However, if joint inflammation (dolor, rubor, calor, tumor) is present or the symptom cannot be produced or explained, an x-ray is mandatory and a referral is suggested.

This basic conservative strategy is justified because of the unusual nature of joint complaints in young patients. X-rays are useful because congenital disorders, tumors, and growth disturbances occur at a much greater frequency in youth and may present with vague symptoms and a normal physical exam. Even trauma that is severe enough to result in soft-tissue swelling may be forceful enough to cause a fracture to the epiphyseal plate or a slipped epiphyses, both of which may lead to future problems if not treated properly.

The term *growing pains* is used most accurately as a description rather than as a diagnosis. The differential diagnosis involves any potential cause of pediatric musculoskeletal pain. True growing pains are defined according to the following criteria and assume that other causes have been systematically excluded:

- leg pain
- aspirin responsive
- children under 8 years old affected
- family history
- not associated with rapid growth spurts
- complaints of pain between joints (not joint pain)
- bilateral pain over time

WHEN TO REFER

For the majority of musculoskeletal problems that present to a physician in a community-based practice, the diagnosis and initial management can be effectively done in the office. There are exceptions and these are generally situations in which greater experience and specialized knowledge are needed to ensure the optimal outcome (see Table 1–6). The primary care physician should refer these

TABLE 1–6. REFERRAL CRITERIA

Undiagnosed synovitis
Failing function
Multisystem disease
Consideration of immunosuppressive, steroid, or disease-modifying agent
Any child with synovitis
Diagnostic arthrocentesis/biopsy
Unresolved symptoms more than 6 weeks
Progressive symptoms or signs

problems on for another opinion, but he or she is still the best person to integrate and execute the advice from the specialist, in most cases.

REFERENCES

Hoppenfeld S: *Physical Examination of the Spine and Extremities.* Appleton-Century-Crafts, New York, 1976. A guide to the musculoskeletal examination with excellent illustrations.

Kelley WN, Harris ED, Ruddy S, Sledge CB (eds): *Textbook of Rheumatology*, 3rd edition. WB Saunders, Philadelphia, 1988. Multiauthored, comprehensive reference. Excellent discussion on surgical options.

McCarty DJ (ed): *Arthritis & Allied Conditions. A Textbook of Rheumatology.* 11th edition. Lea & Febiger, Philadelphia, 1989. Multiauthored, comprehensive reference.

Polley HF, Hunder GG: *Rheumatological Interviewing and Physical Examination of the Joints.* Second edition. WB Saunders, Philadelphia, 1978.

Sheon RP, Moskowitz RW, Goldberg V (eds): *Soft Tissue Rheumatic Pain: Recognition, Management, Prevention.* 2nd edition. Lea & Febiger, Philadelphia, 1987. The most extensive coverage of non-articular rheumatism with excellent literature review on unusual syndromes.

2 Pain in Neck, Shoulder, and Upper Extremity

Like back pain, the majority of neck, shoulder, and arm pain syndromes are due to mechanical causes or soft-tissue lesions. Apart from traumatic conditions, 95% of painful shoulders are the result of degenerative tendinitis and bursitis. Arthritis of the acromioclavicular or glenohumeral joints is uncommon. In this chapter, the common neck, shoulder, and arm pain symptoms are discussed. The management of acute trauma (fractures, dislocation) and pain referred from the heart or gastrointestinal tract are beyond the scope of this chapter. Bone disorders and inflammatory conditions other than tendinitis are discussed briefly in Chapter 4, Low Back Pain. The same points apply to neck pain, although these bone disorders and inflammatory conditions rarely cause neck pain without symptoms in the lower spine.

PHYSIOLOGY OF NECK AND SHOULDER PAIN

Pain in or referred from the neck comes from the irritation of sensitive tissues. The cervical vertebra and the anterior longitudinal ligaments are relatively insensitive tissues. Tumor, infections, or metabolic bone disease of the vertebral bodies produce sensations of deep, vague pain unrelated to motion of the spine. The sensitivity of the intervertebral disc is controversial, but it is devoid of nerve fibers. The posterior longitudinal ligament, the cervical nerve roots, the posterior apophyseal joints, and the neck muscles are pain sensitive.

Purely localized pain is mediated through the branches of the posterior rami of the spinal nerves and cervical plexus.

Pain felt at the shoulder provides little clue to its origin, as any structure in the C5 dermatome may refer pain to the shoulder. The only shoulder structure outside this dermatome is the acromioclavicular joint, which falls in the C4 dermatome. Shoulder and neck pain may result from disorders in the posterior scapular, interscapular, and suspensory muscles, which are mediated through the posterior spinal nerve branches. Shoulder pain from shoulder joint disease is recorded from branches of the brachial plexus. Well-circumscribed pain is localized with a finger and radicular pain is localized with the entire hand. Pain with lancinating qualities, numbness, or tingling should be treated as neurogenic or vascular until proven otherwise.

DIAGNOSTIC STRATEGY

In an ambulatory practice, the goals of diagnosing and managing neck, shoulder, and arm pain are:

1. Exclude treatable causes
2. Control discomfort
3. Prevent physical and psychological disability
4. Prevent recurrences

In sorting out neck pain complaints, one should not miss:

1. Cervical spondylosis with neurological deficits
2. Herniated cervical disc
3. Meningitis
4. Infection of the bone or epidural space
5. Neck pain referral from another source

For shoulder and arm pain, one should not miss:

1. Sympathetic reflex dystrophy syndrome
2. Septic arthritis
3. Acute internal derangement (acute rotator-cuff tear, glenoid labrum tear)
4. Spinal cord tumor
5. Herniated cervical disc

Inflammatory arthritis, tumor, and metabolic bone disease of these regions are "treatable," but earlier treatment is unlikely to improve the ultimate outcome. Moreover, these conditions would eventually be diagnosed by their atypical features, clinical course, and lack of response to therapy. As for most conditions, careful follow-up is the key to successful management.

On the basis of a history, paying attention to the character of the pain and modifying influences, and using the examination to locate the anatomical origin of the pain, the physician can treat it with a minimum of diagnostic studies. Atypical features constitute "red flags" (Table 2–1), suggesting conditions that require more than symptomatic treatment.

TABLE 2–1. NECK PAIN: RED FLAGS

Meningismus
New onset under age 20
Neuromotor deficits
Constitutional symptoms
Neck and shoulder examination normal
Pain not improved by lying down

PHYSICAL EXAMINATION

In the sitting position, the patient is taken through active then passive range of movements to evaluate the neck. Rotating the head is normally possible to 45° bilaterally and involves C1 and C2. Normally, joint motion comes to a soft stop, which is quite distinct from the bone-hard feel of spondylitis or advanced osteoarthritis or the crisp feel of a cervical disc lesion. The patient should be able to put the chin on the chest and look to the ceiling (extension equal to about 40°), laterally flex to 45° (C3–C5). If neck pain is due to muscle spasm in part or in whole, stretching the involved muscle will diminish the pain. When lateral head tilt produces pain in the contralateral cervical muscles, suspect muscle spasm as a primary problem. When lateral head tilt produces ipsilateral neck and shoulder pain, think of a herniated cervical disc.

Myelopathy and peripheral nerve root lesions may be tested with the person sitting. The patient is asked to stick out the tongue to check for fasciculations of the tongue, which point to nerve-root irritation at the occipital-cervical junction. The strength of the deltoids, biceps, and intrinsic muscle of the hands are assessed. The large muscles are tested against resistance to the point of overcoming the subject's strength. Using one, two, or three fingers of the examining hand to resist provides a method of grading muscle power. Elbow flexion and wrist extension tests C6. Elbow extension and wrist flexion tests C7.

The ability to maintain opposition of the thumb tests median-nerve and C6 function. Strength in maintaining opposition of the thumb and little finger tests the ulnar nerve and the C7-T1 root. Finally, the deep tendon reflexes and Babinski's reflex are checked, thus completing the screen for neurological problems.

Checking for cervical muscle spasm is unreliable if it is done with the person erect. In this position the neck muscles are either tense from pain or taut to support the head and, thus, spasm may not be easily appreciated. A better technique is to have the patient supine with the head cradled in the examiner's hand while the other hand palpates for tenderness of the paraspinal muscles, the interspinous ligament, the posterior spines, and the tendinous insertions.

If the neck can be taken through a smooth and painless range of motion, it is almost certainly not the cause of the problem. It is either painful because of referred pain, almost always from the shoulder (and rarely from the mediastinal structures, the heart, the upper airway, or posterior fossa), or from psychological causes. Except for posterior fossa lesions, the other sources of neck pain almost always have associated symptoms that suggest a diagnosis. Likewise, if the patient can smoothly and comfortably lift his or her arms above the head (Figure 2–1), significant pathology of the shoulder is unlikely and the pain must either be referred or of a psychological origin. When injury or disease causes fixation of the gleno- and scapulo-humeral joints, limitation of abduction and of forward flexion occurs, and normal scapulo-humeral rhythm is lost. However, rotation and elevation of the scapula allows elevation of the arm to about 65°, even though no movement takes place between the humerus and the scapula ("shrugging"). If the person has difficulty elevating his or her arms, a detailed

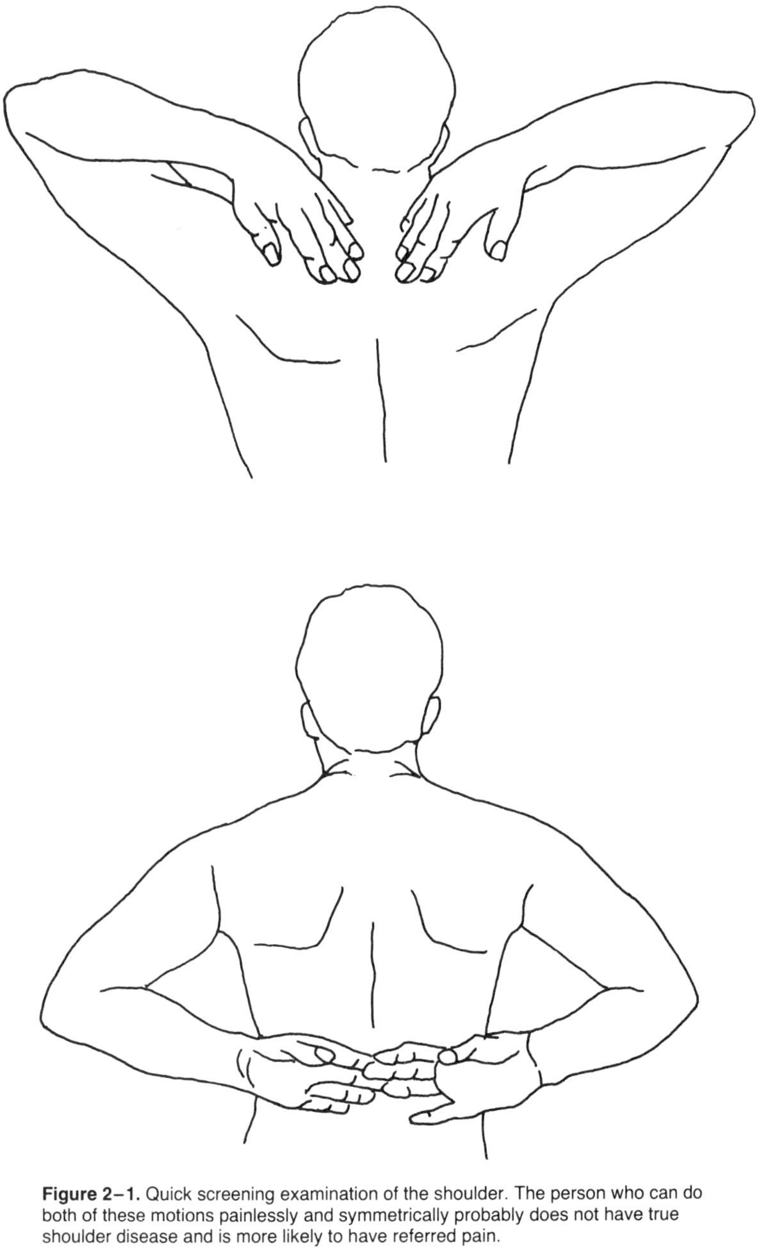

Figure 2–1. Quick screening examination of the shoulder. The person who can do both of these motions painlessly and symmetrically probably does not have true shoulder disease and is more likely to have referred pain.

examination of the shoulder locates the potential sources of pain. The shoulder is taken through abduction, internal and external rotation and forward flexion, first actively then passively. The examiner then searches for areas of point tenderness, which could be tendinitis, bursitis, or muscular trigger points. The subacromial bursa, the bicipital groove, and muscles of the scapula are frequent sites of involvement. Sometimes, an examination may be impossible to complete because of severe muscle spasm or pain. Examine to the extent possible, provide analgesia, and reexamine the person. The follow-up examination is most useful to ensure that the diagnosis has been correct and that management has been successful.

The diagnostic information of radiographs in acute pain symptoms is limited. An abnormal radiograph of the neck or shoulder may be consistent with joint-space infection, osteomyelitis, fracture, tumor, loose body, or extraarticular deposits of calcium, but the absence of specific findings, especially early in the disease process, does not exclude any of these diagnoses. A posterior osteophyte impinging on the spinal cord may not be visible on plain x-ray. Disc lesions occur in radiographically normal areas. On the other hand, the presence of abnormalities does not necessarily mean that they are the cause of the problem. Reduction in one or more disc spaces or loss of the lordotic curve are common findings in asymptomatic individuals. Osteophyte formation is the rule in older patients and usually is not accompanied by any discomfort or functional problem. Minor spondylolisthesis may be seen at the third or fourth cervical vertebra and has no significance.

In one study to establish the diagnostic value of cervical and lumbar spine x-rays, 500 males between the ages of 18 and 65, selected for the absence of significant injuries, rheumatoid arthritis, and systemic illnesses and for unsettled claims or compensation for joint complaints, were examined roentgenographically and clinically by two blinded physicians. The correlation between neck or back pain and roentgenographic findings suggested that the roentgenogram had little value in the individual case and the severity of roentgenographic findings correlated poorly with the severity of symptoms.

Acute shoulder pain is associated with soft-tissue calcifications in one out of three instances, but their presence does not dictate specific treatment or have any prognostic value. Findings such as tubercular irregularities and calcific deposits in tendons and bursa do not correlate with either rotator-cuff degeneration or shoulder pain. Thus, x-ray screening in evaluating shoulder and neck pain is of marginal value when features are typical and the exam is abnormal. X-rays are most likely to be helpful in the following instances:

1. Sudden, severe pain with or without trauma
2. Constitutional symptoms
3. Locking present
4. Failed response to therapy

Neurophysiological studies document cervical radiculopathy by providing an objective measure of nerve damage. With acute nerve impingement, the earliest clinical changes are loss or diminution of deep tendon reflexes. After several

TABLE 2–2. PAIN IN THE UPPER EXTREMITIES

History	Significance
Abrupt onset	Crystal synovitis, internal derangement, fracture
Fever, chills, or rash	Sepsis
Polyarthritis, systemic symptoms	Systemic illness
Inability to use	Internal derangement
Pain awakens from sleep	Structural damage, neurogenic, ischemic
Pain with complete joint rest	Infection, osseous lesion, crystal synovitis
Pain with numbness, tingling, burning, or lancinating quality	Neurovascular compromise
Physical	**Significance**
Effusion	Synovitis (arthritis)
Redness over joint	Infection
Trauma with significant soft tissue damage	Fracture or internal derangement

weeks, up to 6, objective muscle wasting or a decrease in strength are noticed. Nerve conduction testing is used to establish a baseline and to ascertain whether the denervation is acute or chronic. For most cases, if surgical intervention is not a consideration, this documentation does not provide information beyond that of the examination or the patient's symptoms.

In summary, the efficient evaluation of neck, shoulder, and arm pain complaints depends on obtaining a description of the pain, particularly modifying factors; locating the source of pain; excluding treatable conditions; treatment; and follow-up. Cues in the history or physical examination that suggest specific treatable conditions are summarized in Table 2–2.

Neck Pain (Table 2–3)

Neck pain in the primary care setting is almost always from a mechanical, not an inflammatory, cause. Mechanical neck pain, be it due to osteoarthritis or postural strain, is worse at the end of the day, and with active and passive movements, and is relieved by complete rest. Pain or stiffness in the morning suggests an inflammatory component or postural strain during sleep (lying on too many pillows or on one's chest). Pain that interferes with sleep is due to tendinitis, nerve compression, severe muscle spasm, or infection of the bone or disc space. Neck pain complaints without some localizing findings are referred, psychogenic, or due to a lesion of the vertebral body itself (tumor, infection).

Mechanical Neck Pain (Cervical Muscle Spasm)

Pain sensation from muscle is carried by pain fibers in the muscle, particularly at the point of muscle insertion and near the aponeurosis close to bone attachments. The posterior neck muscles are chronically stretched in postural stresses resulting from slumped posture, sloped shoulders, and winged scapula. The dull, aching discomfort is noticeable at rest and at the end of the day, rather

TABLE 2–3. CAUSES OF NECK PAIN

Mechanical

Trauma
- sprain, acute and subacute (whiplash)
- fracture, dislocation
- spasm

Intrinsic
- postural strain

Degenerative
- herniated disc
- osteoarthritis

Osseous

Tumor
- benign (hemangioma, giant-cell tumor, benign chondroblastoma, aneurysm bone cyst, osteoid osteoma, enchondroma, giant-cell tumor)
- malignant (metastic or primary; multiple myeloma, chondroblastoma, chondrosarcoma, Ewing's sarcoma)

Metabolic bone disease
- osteoporosis
- osteomalacia

Infection
- meningitis
- infection of disc space, vertebral body

Soft tissue
- tendinitis
- fibrositis

Arthritis
- spondylitis
- rheumatoid arthritis

Referred

Shoulder
Heart and related structures
Esophagus
Pharynx
Posterior fossae of the brain

Psychological

Hysterial torticullis
Functional
Malingering

than in active use of the muscles — a historical point that is explained by the fact that the sensory fibers in the muscle respond to acute passive stretching but not to active muscle tension. Sustained contraction of the posterior neck muscles from tension, postural strain, or irritative lesions of the neck (such as inflammed nodes) contributes to muscle pain. The physical examination shows localized tenderness over the sternomastoid, trapezius, or paraspinal muscles, and the head may be held uncomfortably with a tilt toward the affected side. Muscle spasm of the cervical spine also occurs with direct injury or from prolonged contraction secondary to inflammation of the muscle or of the cervical lymph nodes.

Tendinitis

Inflammation, presumably from degeneration of tendon fibers at the junction to bone, occurs in the erector spinae tendon (occipital tendinitis), the sternocleidomastoid tendon, or the ligamentum nuchae tendon. The physical examination shows focal tenderness at the insertion site that is aggravated by maneuvers that stretch the tendon.

Occipital tendinitis produces upper neck pain and headache at the occiput that radiates over the back of the head, is most noticeable on awakening, and is followed by stiffness down the shoulder blades. Tenderness in the suboccipital area accentuated by passive resistance to extension confirms the diagnosis.

Tendinitis of the ligamentum nuchae produces intermittent nonprogressive local midcervical discomfort with cracking or clicking, which usually requires special effort to elicit. Well-localized tenderness near the spinous processes makes the diagnosis. On occasion, these are associated with minute calcification.

Sternocleidomastoid tendinitis produces unilateral pain involving the neck, the ear, and the side of the head. A history of trauma or unaccustomed activities may be in the background, but a complete lack of antecedent history is equally common. On examination, a tender and tight sternomastoid is appreciated and tenderness is well localized to the tip of the mastoid process. Motion to the opposite side makes the pain worse and tilting the head to the involved side reduces the pain.

Moderate-to-severe tendinitis responds to rest, time, or local injections of anesthetic and corticosteroids into the area of maximal pain. The natural history of such lesions is variable.

Cervical Osteoarthritis (Cervical Spondylosis)

Osteoarthritis occurs only in the apophyseal joints of the spine and uncovertebral (Luschka) joints of the vertebral bodies. Disc degeneration produces osteophytes of the vertebral bodies, but this is not strictly osteoarthrosis. Degenerative changes in the cervical spine are found almost universally after the age of 50, and one must not automatically attribute all neck and shoulder pain to x-ray changes of osteoarthritis. There is no correlation with either the presence of neck pain or the severity of neck pain and the radiological appearance. Discomfort is more likely to arise from soft-tissue problems.

Degenerative changes of occipitoatlanto and atlantoaxial joints produce upper neck pain without radiation that are related to head rotation. Antecedent trauma or repeated injuries to the suboccipital joint may predispose the joints to degenerative change.

Osteoarthritis of cervical vertebra from C3 to C7 produces aching pain in the neck and shoulder, which is characteristically worse with activity and at the end of the day and is relieved by rest. Pain may also occur from osteophytes or disc protrusion compressing elements of the spinal cord, the spinal roots, the spinal cord itself, and/or the basilar vertebral circulation. These causes of cervical pain are discussed under Neck, Shoulder Pain with Radiation.

Traumatic Injury to the Neck

Whiplash, traumatic cervical syndrome, flexion-extension injury, and acceleration-extension injury denote the syndrome of neck pain due to trauma. *Whiplash* is the common term for injuries in which the head moves forward without direct impact with any object followed by extension of the cervical spine beyond the normal range of motion or rapid lateral flexion limited only by the shoulder followed by flexion in the opposite direction. Neck pain arises from minute tears of cervical muscles and structures, and from muscle spasm.

If a person has pain within 30 minutes of injury, ligaments have been damaged. The pain, usually bilateral, increases in intensity over the next 2 or 3 days. Lateral head tilt produces pain in the contralateral trapezius or sternocleidomastoid muscles that are in spasm.

A second syndrome with identical physical findings develops 24 hours after the injury. On awakening after the accident, the person is unable to move the head or neck. Hemorrhage into the cervical muscles may be responsible. A slower onset of symptoms is associated with a better prognosis.

Cervical trauma may precipitate acute herniation or prolapse of the disc(s), causing symptoms in the neck, shoulder, or upper extremity acutely or days to weeks after the inciting event. When acute neck pain does not get better, consider the possibility of a disc herniation.

Referred Neck Pain

Pain may be referred to the shoulder and/or the base of the neck from a variety of sources. The undersurface of the diaphragm is supplied from the phrenic nerve derived from cervical segments 3, 4, and 5, which also innervates the cutaneous sensation of the neck and shoulder. Thus, irritation of the diaphragm may result in neck and shoulder symptoms.

Central structures in the chest, esophagus, heart, its vessels, and supporting structures may also cause neck pain. Lesions near the center of the diaphragm cause discomfort between the neck and shoulder, whereas lesions near the lateral borders of the diaphragm may be appreciated at the tip of the shoulder.

Pharyngitis may also cause anterior neck pain, but it is unlikely to be missed. Complication such as peritonsillar abscess or retropharyngitis may cause diffuse neck pain from protective splinting of the cervical muscles. Soft-tissue radiographs of the neck are indicated.

TREATMENT OF NECK PAIN

Acute neck pain of mechanical cause gets better. Whether the natural history is improved by any specific "treatment" is untested. The majority of persons with acute neck pain, even those with paresthesias and objective weakness or decreased deep-tendon reflexes, have significant pain relief in 4 to 5 days. Between 70% and 80% of persons will be cured or will have only mild symptoms by 3 to

6 weeks. The treatment of cervical muscle spasm with such agents as diazepam compared to phenobarbital or placebo shows no clearly superior clinical effect.

A primary objective of treatment is patient education on how to minimize stresses to the cervical spine. Patients with neck pain should sit, stand, walk, and lie in a position to flatten the nape of the neck. Postural strain occurs in short individuals who extend their necks to establish eye contact with taller persons, round-shouldered persons whose necks are in exaggerated lordosis, women who are inclined to hold up their chin to eliminate neck wrinkles, and persons who habitually lean on their elbows. Also, workers whose projects are above eye level (car mechanic) and persons with Ben Franklin glasses or bifocal lenses may have neck strain on a similar basis. Persons with neck pain should avoid lying on their stomach as the neck is bent backward and the head is twisted far to one side. In lying on the back, the person should have a pillow that should be of such a thickness that the neck is held level with the rest of the spine so that the occipital ligaments and muscle insertions are not strained. A cylindrical pillow that fits in the nape of the neck or a feather pillow tied in the middle supports the neck in a neutral position. A commercially available cylindrical pillow that is soft in the middle and firm at the ends (Jackson Cervical Comfort pillow) is useful for many individuals. It ensures correct positioning of the neck during sleep.

A soft cervical collar (Thomas collar) provides limited immobilization of the head or neck, restricting 5% to 10% of flexion extension, lateral bending, and rotation. Its assets are its minimal expense and comfort. With the first occurrence of neck pain, a medium-sized bath towel folded into a strip whose width is sufficient to flatten the neck's lordosis substitutes nicely for a soft cervical collar. With severe neck pain, recurrent or with radicular symptoms, a firm collar or two soft collars in a pinch effectively splints the cervical spine.

Specific exercises stretch the strong posterior neck muscles and strengthen the anterior muscles. The simplest exercise is done with the person supine. The head is raised slowly off the pillow until it is as close to the chest as possible. The muscles should then be relaxed slowly, allowing the head to gently settle back onto the pillow. One should work up to doing this 20 times a day after gradual graded effort. Analgesics and sedation will be discussed.

Cervical Traction

Cervical traction has enthusiastic supporters and skeptical critics. Some claim that 70% of patients respond to this approach. Since the equipment is relatively inexpensive, can do little harm, and can be used at home, it is worth trying in difficult cases.

Weights of 10 to 15 pounds are used initially and are gradually increased to tolerance. Separation of the cervical vertebrae require 25 to 35 pounds of traction, but many patients are unable to tolerate this.

With acute injuries or severe symptoms, the neck should be splinted and rested. The only proper way to rest the neck is to take the weight of the head off

TABLE 2–4. SHOULDER PAIN SYNDROMES

Acute, Abnormal Exam*
Calcific tendinitis or bursitis
Dislocation
Rotator-cuff tear
Inflammatory arthritis
Infection

Subacute/Chronic, Abnormal Exam*
Supraspinatus tendinitis
Adhesive capsulitis
Rotator-cuff tear
Inflammatory arthritis

Acute or Chronic, Normal Exam*
Referred
Fibrositis
Neurovascular syndromes
Sympathetic reflex dystrophy

* Passive range of motion, resisted abduction, point of maximal tenderness, crepitus

of the neck, and the only way to accomplish this is with bed rest on an as needed basis.

Do not give undue emphasis to therapeutic measures. The measures are meant to make the patient more comfortable, not cure the malady. When symptoms are severe enough to require bed rest, chances are high that the symptoms will persist, though to a lesser degree, for at least 6 weeks and up to 6 months to a year. If the patient is told that the pain will gradually stop, his or her ability to tolerate pain is buttressed. Nevertheless, the patient should be encouraged with a firm and explicit program of increasing daily activity.

Patients with prolonged pain symptoms must be followed closely for latent depression and regression to dependent styles. Helping individuals to live within the limits of their symptoms requires skill. Being firm without reinforcing sick role behavior and listening when catharsis and sympathy are needed are keys to managing acute problems effectively. Persistent pain and/or loss of functional capacity call for a referral.

SHOULDER PAIN

Shoulder pain may be approached initially by determining whether the pain is associated with an abnormal shoulder examination or a normal examination (Table 2–4). If the shoulder exam is abnormal, conservative symptomatic treatment is instituted and the person is reexamined within 2 weeks to ensure that the episode has resolved successfully — that shoulder movements are full. If pain persists despite analgesic/antiinflammatory agents and the maximum of three intraarticular injections, the diagnostic possibilities are limited to rotator-cuff tear, tumor, loose body, glenohumeral arthritis, glenoid labrum tear, and acromioclavicular arthritis.

Shoulder pain with a normal examination of the shoulder suggests a referred source, most often the neck, but occasionally the heart and lungs or from upper abdominal viscera causing diaphramatic irritation.

SHOULDER PAIN WITH ABNORMAL EXAMINATION (BURSITIS/TENDINITIS)

Degeneration of the rotator cuff or tendinitis is the substrate of almost all early persistent shoulder disability. The degenerative process may involve the musculotendinous cuff, the bicipital tendon, or both.

Tendinitis of the shoulder produces discomfort, which is accurately localized by the patient. The course begins with discomfort on lifting the arm, and progresses over weeks to the point where even minimal movements cause unusual pain. This makes the person apprehensive and, eventually, even sleep is interrupted. Tendinitis/bursitis, nerve compression, and severe cartilage destruction are three causes of shoulder pain that can awaken a patient from a sound sleep.

In tendinitis, examination shows a painful arc when the arm is lifted and rotated externally, as the head of the humerus comes into contact with the acromial arch, the motion of a right-hand turn signal. In contrast, true intra-articular glenohumeral pain is made worse by internal rotation, the motion of a left-hand turn signal. In tendinitis, shoulder motion is limited by pain. Active movement is done with trepidation and hesitation. The patient may feel crepitus, cracking, slipping, or soft grinding as the arm is limited. If pain and limitation occur after the arm has been abducted to 90°, then the acromioclavicular joint is involved. With time, any cause of chronic shoulder pain will result in atrophy of the supraspinatus and infraspinatus muscles, and restriction of normal mobility.

Palpation of the shoulder reveals diffuse tenderness over the upper end of the humerus over the cuff, but not the exquisite point tenderness that occurs with bicipital tendinitis or supraspinatus tendinitis with calcification. Figure 2–2 shows the location of the subdeltoid or subacromial bursa along with the other bursae of the shoulder region. Prolonged pain frequently radiates to the posterior shoulder, neck, or elbow. Acute, severe shoulder pain unrelated to trauma is almost always due to tenditinis/subdeltoid bursitis, a condition with pain that crescendos rapidly over a night or several days and brings persons in early for treatment. They are extremely uncomfortable. Few can sleep. The slightest movement of the shoulder produces spasms of pain, and attempts to exercise the shoulder are usually thwarted by protestations of pain. Occasionally, a low-grade fever may be present.

Although calcium hydroxyapatite crystals in the periarticular tissues is the presumed cause of acute subdeltoid bursitis, deposits may be found in 8% of persons over 30 years old without pain. An identical clinical course occurs in the absence of radiographically demonstrated concretions. The shape and location of such deposits does not appear to have a significant bearing on the prognosis.

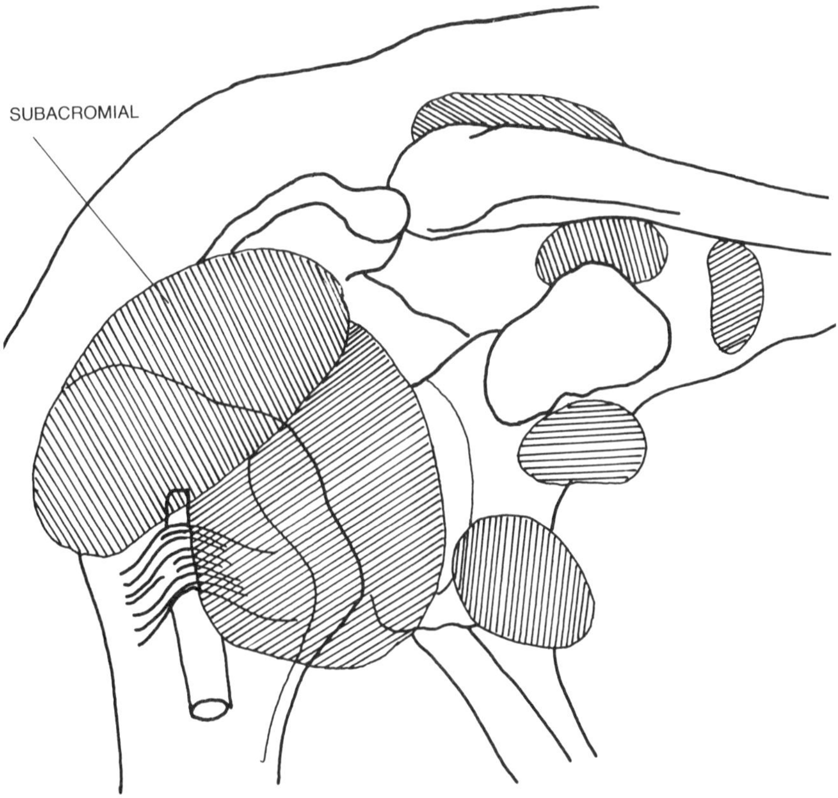

Figure 2–2. Bursae of the shoulder. Of the bursae around the shoulder, the subacromial or subdeltoid bursa is most commonly involved in both acute and chronic bursitis.

Periarticular deposits occur as a result of local changes in the cuff tendons, most commonly, the supraspinatus tendon. During normal arm elevation and abduction, the humeral head is repeatedly depressed downward against the glenoid fossa. Over time, collagen fibers in the tendon break down and calcium phosphate debris accumulate in the tendon. If the debris remains within the tendon, the shoulder is painless and unrestricted. If the deposit ruptures into the bursa sac, acute inflammation and pain ensue, resulting in the clinical syndrome of calcific tendinitis or subacromial bursitis. In this syndrome, the pain comes on rapidly and is fairly acute (a "boil" of the shoulder), preventing normal sleep and function. Although precise clinical differentiation from supraspinatus tendinitis is not always clear nor essential for proper management, supraspinatus tendinitis is associated with a more gradual onset and subacute discomfort.

Bicipital Tendinitis

The long head of the biceps tendon is affected by all movements of the humerus on the scapula and anchors the powerful biceps muscle. It suffers stress from everyday activities, but particularly, overhead work and against force resistance with the arm extended. Inflammation of the synovial sheath of the tendon of the biceps muscle and tissues contiguous to the tendon results from repeated strain or trauma in susceptible individuals. The inflammatory process produces a serofibrinous exudate, eventually leading to a fibrinous mass of adhesions between the tendon, the sheath, and the bicipital groove. An abnormally shallow or roughened bicipital groove may predispose individuals to inflammation.

On examination, the shoulder movements are limited somewhat, but the chief finding is tenderness of the bicipital tendon. In acute cases, persons will have pain on resisted flexion and supination of the forearm (Yergason's sign). In subacute or chronic cases, this physical sign may be absent in up to half of the persons examined.

Bicipital tendinitis and tenosynovitis responds to conservative management consisting of arm rest (a sling), nonsteroidal antiinflammatory agents, or, in cases of severe pain, infiltration with a local anesthetic and/or corticosteroids. If the signs and symptoms persist or increase, consider a rupture or partial rupture of the tendon, of the ligament roof of the bicipital groove, or of the transverse humeral ligament. The critical test for disruption of the transverse humeral ligament is to rotate the arm with the elbow held in flexion. In this maneuver, the examiner's finger in the bicipital groove appreciates the tendon slipping back and forth underneath.

Bicipital tendon rupture is recognized on examination by an abnormal contour of the upper arm (not always obvious), pain in the bicipital groove, and a relaxed biceps muscle on flexion of the elbow.

Rotator-Cuff Tears

The rotator cuff, comprised of the muscles and their tendons (subscapularis, supraspinatus, infraspinatus, and teres minor) that fuse with the joint capsule about one-half inch from its distal margin, provides the fine adjustment in all movements of the humerus, rotates the humerus, and fixes the head of the humerus on the glenoid fossa. The rotators of the shoulder and their connective tissue webbing take the brunt of gross trauma and microtrauma. Rotator-cuff tears occur commonly but are frequently unrecognized. The history and physical examination make the diagnosis likely and an arthrogram establishes the diagnosis.

A person with a tear may give a history of symptoms precipitated by sharp trauma such as a sudden strain in abduction, a blow, or a fall, but the history is not necessary for diagnosis. Indeed, even reaching may tear the cuff, and it is not until some time later that pain, weakness, and restricted movements occur. The quality of pain is worsened by an attempt to elevate the arm above shoulder level. In later stages, pain extends to the deltoid insertion and shoulder-neck angle.

On examination, the patient is unable to raise his or her arm. There is tenderness over the tip of the acromion, crepitus over the shoulder on abduction, and hesitant painful scapulohumeral rhythm. The patient may be unable to initiate abduction. If helped, the arm goes through a weak, painful motion through 70° to 90° of abduction as the tear impinges on the acromion and then decreased pain as the arm is lifted above shoulder level, the so-called painful arc or impingement. The arm can be lowered smoothly and without pain to 90° and then it falls suddenly with pain. ("drop-arm sign")

The cardinal sign of rotator-cuff rupture, persistent weakness, differentiates a tear from chronic tendinitis. Although a person with a significant tear may be able to lift the arm above shoulder height, any amount of resistance will usually prevent abduction. Atrophy of the supraspinatus and infraspinatus, and flattening of the deltoid mass occurs months after a tear.

A torn cuff is almost always tender to palpation. The zone most frequently involved is covered by the corocoacromial arch when the shoulder is in the resting position. This area is palpated by extending the person's shoulder and arm, and pushing the head of the humerus forward.

Treatment of rotator-cuff tears

If a cuff tear is small or long-standing, conservative management is indicated. If the tear is of recent onset (i.e., less than 2 months) or large, conservative treatment still consists of active shoulder movement within the limits of pain and adequate analgesia to extend this limit, but the patient should be referred to an orthopedic surgeon.

Isometric exercises for the shoulder muscles and advice on how to minimize shoulder stress are essential. The key to maintaining or regaining shoulder function is to improve flexion rather than abduction. If there is no improvement after 6 weeks of conservative management, consider surgery. Massive rotator-cuff ruptures are easily suspected and diagnosed and should be surgically repaired as soon as possible. Delay makes the surgery more difficult and chances an unsatisfactory result.

Acromioclavicular (AC) Arthritis

(Acromioclavicular) arthritis, most commonly post-traumatic, produces pain on the shoulder and the diagnosis is obvious on clinical grounds alone. Sharp pain is noticed after the arm is elevated to 90° and with passive flexing of the arm across the chest at a right angle. The joint line is tender and crepitant on movement. Acute pain is reproduced by pressure over the clavicle with one hand and pushing up on the elbow with the other, thereby moving the two bones against one another.

FROZEN SHOULDER (ADHESIVE CAPSULITIS)

Frozen shoulder — an uncomfortable stiff shoulder that has lost its fluid movements — is the wretched end stage of a variety of shoulder problems. It results from any cause of shoulder pain or prolonged restriction of shoulder movement and, thus, could be prevented if the primary conditions were managed properly, and shoulder mobility and muscle strength were maintained. Older persons, women, and patients with insulin-dependent diabetes are more susceptible, and even a relatively mild disturbance may end as a frozen shoulder.

The condition itself is easily recognized, although the primary event may be elusive. The typical patient is over 50, female, and has had a history of shoulder difficulty for weeks to months, which has progressed to a painful stiffening. The shoulder has lost its normal scapulohumeral rhythm, and the person must shrug in order to lift his or her arm.

Examination shows absent glenohumeral motion, limited abduction, and atrophy of the muscles about the shoulder. An arthrogram shows a contracted joint capsule.

The Reflex Sympathetic Dystrophy Syndrome (RSDS)

The reflex sympathetic dystrophy syndrome or "shoulder-hand syndrome" is an unusual but important symptom complex that occurs in the company of a painful and/or stiff shoulder. One cannot afford to miss this syndrome. Recognized early, it is usually successfully treated; diagnosed in its chronic stage when dystrophic changes and contractures have set in, rehabilitation is slow and difficult. A typical patient is over 50 years old and has a history of precipitants, such as myocardial infarction; trauma; spinal disc disease preceding or accompanying the involvement of the hand by pain, swelling, and vasomotor instability phenomena (Raynaud's phenomenon, mottling, color changes, excess sweating); and, later on, trophic changes, including skin and muscle atrophy, pigmentary changes, hypertrichosis, and nail changes. Early on, pain out of proportion to the physical findings is the cardinal feature of the syndrome. Frequently, there is radiological evidence of severe, patchy osteoporosis, which gives the bone the appearance of being moth-eaten. This radiographic picture has been called Sudek's atrophy. The shoulder or hand or fingers may be affected in some circumscribed cases. Rarely, the feet can have a similar involvement.

Symptoms may arise suddenly with pain and stiffness of the shoulder followed shortly by swelling, vasomotor changes, and hyperesthesia and disability of the hand. These symptoms will follow quickly after a precipitating event or in weeks or months after the event.

In the first stage of the syndrome, a full-blown shoulder and hand involvement often lasts 3 to 6 months. Subsequently, partial or complete resolution of the swelling occurs, and vasomotor disturbance, early trophic changes, and contractures may appear. This phase may last 3 to 6 months. The third stage, the end stage, is dominated by atrophy or dystrophy of the fingers and hands, blurring of the skin creases of the dorsum hand, contractures of the fingers in flexion, and occasionally a frozen shoulder as well. All the stages can be telescoped within a short time in the occasional patient. Radiographic changes occur throughout the clinical course, although indistinct in the early stages. The opposite shoulder or hand is usually involved, although not clinically, and provides evidence for a central neural mechanism. All or parts of the clinical syndrome may undergo spontaneous resolution at any time. Systemic symptoms do not occur and if present suggest other diagnoses. The sedimentation rate may be increased in a quarter of the patients, but usually for other reasons.

The severity of the syndrome is not proportional to the extent of the provocative condition nor the physical findings. Mild and uneventful myocardial infarction may be followed by the most troublesome and protracted reflex syndrome, or minor trauma may induce severe pain and dystrophy.

The management of reflex sympathetic dystraphy syndrome is based on active and aggressive physical therapy to ensure a continued range of motion of the shoulder, adequate analgesia, and either systemic steroids and/or stellate ganglion blockade. Sympathetic blocks are comparable to the results from corticosteroids in similar series of patients. Complete recovery or major improvement in pain, swelling, and other signs, and complete or marked recovery of function has been reported in one-third to one-half of patients treated in the early stage, and another one-quarter or one-half have had appreciable benefit in either pain relief or increased function. Follow-up studies show few recurrences and only minor complaints in those patients who have recovered.

Systemic corticosteroids are given in a dose of prednisone, 1 mg/kg, in divided doses given daily for up to 2 weeks and then tapered over a 2-week period to 5 mg each day or 5 to 10 mg every other day. If there is any contraindication to the use of steroids, stellate ganglion blocks should be employed.

Contraindications to stellate blocks are hypersensitivity to procaine or related compounds. If four successive blocks do not show any improvement, more attempts are usually futile. An average of seven, and as many as 14, blocks have been given.

In patients with end-stage reflex sympathetic dystrophy syndrome, only refractory pain justifies the use of these measures. A comprehensive rehabilitation program of exercises provides the most useful approach to overcome disability. For patients with severe functional impairment and irreversible contractures, surgery might be considered.

TREATMENT OF SHOULDER PAIN

The goals of managing acute and subacute shoulder pain are to control pain and to prevent contractures (frozen shoulder) and, possibly, reflex sympathetic dystrophy syndrome. These goals are accomplished by physical modalities, medication, and, in certain circumstances, steroid injection. If pain or the range of motion does not improve, a large rotator-cuff tear, referred pain, impingement syndrome, or adhesive capsulitis are possibilities. The patient should be thoroughly reevaluated, and diagnostic arthroscopy, computed axial tomography scan, or NMRI studies should be considered.

During the acute phase, putting the shoulder to rest with a sling reduces irritation to the joint. Ice packs are applied during the acute phase, which lasts approximately 2 days. Heat theoretically increases the blood flow to inflammed tissues, whereas ice decreases spasm, has local cutaneous anesthetic effects, and may reduce the amount of blood flow to the area.

Prolonged immobilization of the shoulder leads to adhesive capsulitis or frozen shoulder. Even a normal shoulder immobilized for a period of weeks will become stiff with a decreased range of motion.

To prevent contractures, active range of motion exercises within the person's limit of pain should be instituted within the first 4 to 7 days. Codman exercise (pendular exercise) adds traction to the glenohumeral joint, stretches the capsule, and avoids active abduction — a painful maneuver. With the hips flexed, the person dangles the arm holding a weight (either an iron or a 5- to 10-pound bag of rice). Pendular motion is started in a lateral medial plane, in a saggital plane forward and backward, and then in gradually increasing circles. Another program consists of walking one's outstretched arm and fingers up a wall to the limit of pain. Frequent repetitions of both of these exercises ensures that the shoulder will be supple after the acute painful stage has been weathered.

There is no evidence that any analgesia or analgesic/antiinflammatory agent is superior to any other. Based on the pathology of tendinitis and bursitis, the major cause of shoulder pain, antiinflammatory drugs are recommended. For mild-to-moderate symptoms that occur in subacute or chronic shoulder pain, aspirin suffices. Phenylbutazone, one of the most potent nonsteroidal antiinflammatory agents, is used but is not indicated, because the drug carries a risk of marrow aplasia. For acute severe pain, local injection of corticosteroid and an anesthetic agent relieves the symptoms effectively.

However, the efficacy of intraarticular corticosteroids in the treatment of painful shoulders is by no means settled. Early studies, many uncontrolled, with conflicting results looked at a heterogeneous group of painful shoulder syndromes and a variety of injection techniques, each claiming to be superior. Objective and subjective improvements were poorly documented.

A study compared steroids with placebo injection in the painful shoulder. One hundred and one consecutive patients were studied with a) pain on resisted abduction and/or external rotation of the arm, and/or b) loss of passive movement(s) of the glenohumeral joint. Diagnostic exclusions were polymyalgia rheumatica, biceps tendinitis, polyarthritis with involvement of the shoulder joint, abnormal neurological signs, or the shoulder/hand syndrome, and any possible association with a cerebrovascular accident, cardiac ischemia, herpes zoster, and arthritis of the acromioclavicular joint. All patients were given analgesics and injections of prednisolone acetate or of normal saline on the first visit and at 2 weeks according to a random treatment allocation schedule. Injections were done posteriorly into the subdeltoid bursa and the glenohumeral joint. Arthrograms indicated that injections into the subacromial bursa were readily accomplished, but those into the joint were done inconstantly.

In the rotator-cuff/capsulitis group of lesions, local steroid injection produced a statistically significant improvement in passive shoulder movement, compared with controls, and a trend towards reduction of pain on resisted movements. Benefits were most marked in patients with rotator-cuff lesions who showed relatively more pain on resisted movement and had less severe loss of passive movement. Factors such as the duration of symptoms, x-ray changes, or previous trauma to the shoulder did not affect the response to steroid injections.

In a single-blind trial comparing acupuncture, steroid injections, tolmetin, and ultrasound with placebo pills in various combinations in 60 patients with rotator-cuff lesions for over 4 weeks, little difference could be found among the regimens.

Similarly, in 42 patients with frozen shoulders followed for 8 months, all of whom participated in exercises, the long-term advantages between intraarticular steroids, mobilization, ice, and no treatment were minimal, although steroids seemed to be the best for improving the range of motion and reducing pain early on in the course of the disease.

The same group compared patients with frozen shoulder randomly assigned to prednisone 10 mg a day for a month followed by 5 mg a day for 2 weeks with patients receiving no specific treatment. Early on, the steroid-treated group fared better, but at 8 months the differences were lost.

In 40 patients with *acute* rotator-cuff tendinitis, randomly assigned to subacromial injections of triamcinolone (40 mg) or to oral indomethacin (100 mg/day) in a double-blind study, no differences could be discerned at 6 weeks.

The latest study involving a variety of patients with chronic and acute shoulder pain was a randomized, double-blind study comparing placebo, triamcinolone subacromial bursa injection, and naproxen. At 2 and 4 weeks, the steroid injection was found to be superior to naproxen; both were better than placebo. Patients who were worst at onset improved the most.

Therefore, the data indicates that acutely painful shoulders from a variety of causes with the worst pain and range of motion are helped by steroids in the short term, whereas chronically painful shoulders with limitations of range of motion respond less well. Over the extended period, no medical treatment is clearly better, but steroid injection reduces the total amount of pain and disability.

PATIENT EDUCATION

Learning new patterns of shoulder use to protect the joint from daily trauma is necessary to avoid further trauma. The patient should face the object being handled, keeping the elbows in front and below shoulder level. To minimize leverage on the shoulder, heavy objects should be held as close to the body as possible. Supporting the weight of the arm minimizes impingement and can be accomplished by using chair arms at the proper height and positioning work below shoulder level close to the body. In shoulder pain of less than 2 weeks duration, or in which some movement has been maintained, there is no evidence to suggest that strengthening the shoulder musculature is necessary. However, when shoulder use has been restricted beyond this period, therapeutic exercises to maintain muscle tone should be advised.

SHOULDER/NECK PAIN WITH RADIATION

Conditions that produce shoulder discomfort and arm pain include:

- spinal cord tumor
- nerve root or spinal cord compression
- thoracic outlet syndrome

All are potential surgical problems. In this group of disorders, pain radiates below the elbow to the forearm or hand, and not just to the deltoid insertion, the usual radiation of primary shoulder conditions. The pain is characteristically neurogenic or ischemic. Neurogenic pain is tingling, lancinating, numb or burning, and usually involves a specific dermatome. Vascular pain is localized to the entire forearm or entire hand, and is appreciated as fullness or a bursting sensation; occasionally transient pins and needles; discoloration; and in severe vascular obstruction, decreased sensation and claudication. Occasionally, muscular pain originating in the posterior scapular region may radiate down the posterior arm and dorsum of the forearm to the fourth and fifth fingers.

In nerve-root compression, neck bending or twisting triggers symptoms, and recumbency relieves symptoms. Sleep often precipitates pain from vascular sources. Work done above shoulder level frequently aggravates the pain of neurovascular compression syndromes.

CERVICAL NERVE-ROOT COMPRESSION SYNDROMES

Disc Lesions

Nerve-root compression most commonly results from disc lesions. Normally, the nerve root occupies one third of the foramen, thus considerable encroachment by disc and/or bone spur is necessary to produce compression. An acute herniated cervical disc usually comes after a clear-cut injury, (a vertebral compression injury, such as a fall) or after a severe voluntary muscular contraction (such as lifting a heavy object).

Acute nerve-root compression produces pain, then numbness and tingling, starting in the shoulder and quickly peaking over hours, radiating to the upper arm, forearm, and fingers. Usually involving one nerve root, the pain radiation pattern points to the culpable nerve root, most commonly at the C5–C6 level with the C4–C5 and C6–C7 levels equally prevalent thereafter. Sixth root compression causes thumb and index finger symptoms, the seventh gets the middle finger, and the eighth root affects the fourth and fifth fingers. Pressure on the sixth and seventh nerve roots may actually mimic coronary insufficiency. Moving the neck makes the pain worse, and the person learns to limit his or her movements.

Weakness follows pain in short order, the pattern depending on the particular nerve root involved (Table 2–5). Weakness and atrophy of the biceps and deltoids implicates the space between C5 and C6; of the triceps, the C6–C7 area; and of the small muscles of the hand, the eighth cervical root. Motor deficits are more reliable than sensory changes to locate the lesion.

An insidious onset occurs much more commonly, beginning with neck ache, extending eventually to the shoulder, forearm, and hand. The course may be interrupted by flare-ups, but the pattern is one of indolent progression.

The examination shows restricted neck movements — difficulty touching one's chin to the chest and looking to the ceiling. Tilting the head to the side of the lesion reproduces the pain and makes it worse, and tilting away decreases discomfort.

Acute attacks of radicular pain in persons without degenerative disease of the cervical spine or trauma should be treated as an acute herniated disc. A disc may also compress the spinal cord, in which case weakness with or without stiffness of one or both legs occurs in over 90% of persons. These cases should be followed with a neurosurgeon.

Other presentations of cervical disc herniation are paresthesias in one or both hands; root pain referred to the neck, shoulders, or arms; or electric shock sensation on turning or flexing the head. Significant urinary symptoms are uncommon. The physical examination shows upper motor neuron signs in the lower limbs, coupled with lower motor neuron findings in the arms. Sensory loss occurs uncommonly in the lower limbs.

Spinal Cord Compression

The clinical features of cervical myelopathy are extremely variable. In many cases, it is difficult to relate the full clinical picture to the observed abnormalities in the cervical spine. The most common site for intervertebral disc protrusion is at the C5–C6 level, with the C4–C5 and C6–C7 levels equally affected thereafter. Typical symptoms occur in one or both legs — weakness with or without stiffness is present in over 90% of patients at the time of diagnosis. A common complaint is, "Doctor, my foot's dragging." The second most common presenting symptoms is paresthesia (*but not pain*) in one or both hands. Occasionally, patients complain of root pains and these may be referred to the neck, shoulders, or arms. Some patients complain of an electric shock sensation on turning or flexing the head. Significant urinary symptoms are uncommon.

The typical physical findings are an upper motor neuron lesion in the lower limbs, coupled with lower motor neuron findings in the arms. Sensory loss may occur, but this is uncommon in the lower limbs.

As in the lower back, an abnormally narrow spinal canal from a congenital lesion, osteophytes, or vertebral body subluxation or disc may produce neck and upper limb discomfort followed by lower limb functional impairment. Three quarters of the patients are over age 65. The cardinal sign of myelopathy is upper motor neuron disease of the lower extremity, spastic pathological reflexes and weakness, and weakness or atrophy of the upper limbs. The diagnosis is

TABLE 2–5. CLINICAL FINDINGS IN THE COMMON CERVICAL RADICULAR SYNDROMES

	Usual Distribution of Pain	Principally Affected Muscles	Sensory Loss	Deep Tendon Reflexes
C6	Neck, parascapular, lateral aspect of arm and forearm	Biceps, brachioradialis, wrist extensors and flexors	Radial border of forearm, thumb	Biceps and/or brachioradialis diminished
C7	Neck, parascapular, posterolateral arm, dorsum of forearm	Triceps, wrist, finger flexors and extensors	Dorsum of forearm; index and middle fingers	Triceps diminished

suspected on clinical examination and is confirmed by a myelogram, computed tomography scan, or magnetic resonance imaging studies.

Conservative management of neck pain should be carried out initially. If significant cervical stenosis exists, traction may not only be ineffectual, but may make the person worse. Persistent or important neurological deficits indicate the need for surgery. Of the techniques used to document the root lesion, the clinical examination and electromyography are the most accurate. The cervical myelogram is apt to show a posterior cervical disc protrusion in many persons over age 30, no matter what symptoms or signs may be present. Large defects of any shape with or without compression may be asymptomatic. Myelography is used as a preoperative test to guide the surgeon's approach and to exclude other cord lesions such as spinal-cord tumors (neuromas and meningiomas).

Tumors of the Spinal Cord

Cervical cord tumors are rare but curable if surgery is done before the tumor has spread and permanent nerve damage has occurred. Fortunately, many primary tumors of the cord have low invasive potential and tend to be well delineated, a good situation for surgical cure. Profound motor and sensory deficits with persistent and bilateral pain should raise the possibility. Persons characteristically complain of pain that does not allow them to find a comfortable position.

TREATMENT OF NECK PAIN

Acute sudden severe neck pain with radicular symptoms in patients who have had no prior history of degenerative disease of the cervical spine should be treated as if there was an acute herniated disc and should be referred to a neurosurgeon. Likewise, patients with suspected vertebral basilar insufficiency (i.e., with symptoms of positional dizziness, vertigo, tinnitus, diplopia, dysarthria, dysphagia, unilateral or bilateral weakness of the arm or leg associated with numbness or tingling in one or both sides of the body, loss of hearing with ataxia, signs of cerebellar dysfunction, drop attacks, stroke, etc.) should be referred to a neurosurgeon.

For subacute and chronic pain or acute exacerbations with a chronic history, resting the neck in a proper position is essential. Local measures to reduce muscle spasm, such as stretching or heat or cold applications, are also helpful, as muscle spasm plays a strong role in the genesis of pain. Cervical collars may help splint the neck and minimize trauma.

A variety of collars are available. The most effective and expensive are rigid collars that enclose the neck, but these are poorly tolerated. A comfortable, inexpensive substitute can be made with a hand towel rolled into a 4″ to 6″ rope. In a collar, it is vital that the neck be maintained in a position to minimize hyperextension. Commonly used soft collars do not restrict the motion of the spine.

When a collar is used, additional measures are needed at night. A cylinder pillow in the nape of the neck or a feather pillow tied in the middle are useful aids to support the neck in a proper position. The cervical spine should be held level with the rest of the spine.

Analgesics may be required for a short time to provide comfort. Short courses of sedation are helpful to maintain bed rest and to relieve muscle spasm. Oral muscle relaxants have never been shown to affect muscle spasm in any convincing manner. Such widely advertised agents as methocarbamol (Robaxin®) have never been demonstrated to be better than placebo alone. Diazepam is slightly better than these agents, but is no better than aspirin. The primary benefit of muscle relaxants, if any, would appear to be their general sedative effect rather than their effect on specific muscle tension.

CERVICAL NEUROVASCULAR COMPRESSION SYNDROME (THORACIC OUTLET SYNDROMES)

The neurovascular bundle of the subclavian artery and vein and the brachial plexus may be compressed at several points along its course, producing signs or symptoms of nerve-root pain or vascular insufficiency. There syndromes are rare and the clinical features include pain, paresthesias, numbness, weakness, discoloration, swelling, and ischemic symptoms or signs ranging from Raynaud's phenomenon to ulceration and gangrene. Potential trouble spots where pinching of the neurovascular bundle may occur are:

1. The triangle between the anterior portion of the scalene muscle (scalene anticus) and the posterior portion (scalene medius);
2. The costoclavicular space bounded by the clavicle, subclavius muscle, first rib, scalene muscle, and scapula; and
3. The axilla, including the pectoralis minor and the median nerve that embraces the axillary artery.

In addition to these anatomical substrates, other factors contribute to symptoms. Positioning may change the relative position of structures, resulting in compression or impingement of vessels and nerves. For instance, when the arm is fully abducted above the head, the axillary artery is pulled across the coracoid process and the head of the humerus. Muscular hypertrophy may reduce the space through which the artery, vein, and nerve must cross.

Congenital variants such as cervical rib, bifid clavicle, and fascial bands behind the scalenus anticus or abnormal insertion of the scalenus medius on the first rib may press on the vessels or nerves when the arm is in certain positions. Traumatic factors such as a previous fracture or dislocation of the humeral head may result in compression. In some cases, these factors may be less important than the presence or absence of arteriosclerotic vessels.

Cervical Rib, Scalenus-Anticus, and Costoclavicular Syndromes

These syndromes are diagnosed on the basis of suspicious symptoms and the physical examination. The Adson (scalene) maneuver decreases the interscalene space, worsening existing compression of the subclavian artery and the C8 and T1 components of the brachial plexus. The subject is instructed to stand at attention in an exaggerated military stance with the shoulder drawn back. The examiner holds the subject's extended arm and palpates for diminution or obliteration of the pulse volume.

Neurovascular compression in the area of the costoclavicular space is suggested if this sign is present, but many normal individuals may have this physical finding with no symptoms. Next, the patient is asked to relax his or her stance, take and hold a deep breath, and then look toward and away from the symptomatic side. If these maneuvers (the Adson or scalene maneuver) diminish or obliterate the radial pulse, compression of the subclavian artery and brachial plexus is suggested, but the absence of the sign does not exclude compression elsewhere.

Hyperabduction Syndrome

Repeated or prolonged hyperabduction of the arms above the head with the elbows flexed in a habit of sleep or occupation (auto mechanics, painters) produces neurovascular symptoms. At two spots, beneath the tendon of the pectoralis muscle and under the coracoid process, compression may occur.

Not all symptoms of neurovascular pain are due to compression syndromes. A herniated cervical disc, cervical spondylosis, and cord tumors may impinge on nerve roots and confuse the picture. A helpful clinical clue is that compression syndromes are usually confined to the C8 nerve root (which supplies the posterior aspect of the arm below the axillary crease, the central part of the palm, and a narrow area on the anterior aspect of the forearm) and the T1 nerve root (the ulnar aspect of the forearm, hand, and little finger). A herniated cervical disc, on the other hand, usually involves the C5 or C6 nerve root, and cervical arthritis involves multiple nerve roots.

These common thoracic outlet syndromes are managed by reassuring the person and educating him regarding positions that cause symptoms. If there is disability, or if ischemic signs exist, a surgical opinion is indicated.

ELBOW PAIN

In the primary care setting, pain in the elbow is usually related to injuries in the form of contusions, sprains and fractures, olecranon bursitis, or epicondylitis. In young children, a common cause is a pulled elbow. Rheumatoid arthritis, the most common rheumatic disease that affects the elbow and other forms of inflammatory arthritis, can be excluded if there is no limitation of the range of motion or synovitis.

Contusions resulting from a direct blow to the elbow usually respond to ice at the time of injury and to rest with gradual resumption of activities as tolerated. One exception is traumatic olecranon bursitis, which many feel should be treated by aspiration followed by compressive dressings for several days.

Sprains of the capsular and ligamentous structures about the elbow commonly involve hyperextension of the valgus mechanism, placing stress on the anterior and medial structures. Sprains are associated with pain and tenderness of the involved ligaments. Check for ligamentous laxity to detect medial or lateral collateral ligament involvement. Management is determined by the degree of injury. In hyperextension and medial collateral ligament sprains, the most common injuries, treatment is conservative. Ice is used immediately, and active range of motion exercises are followed by progressive resistance exercises when the range of motion has returned to normal. For sprains of moderate severity where there is no significant laxity, the elbow is immobilized for 1 to 2 weeks in a splint or a sling.

Olecranon Bursitis

Olecranon bursitis is diagnosed by inspection as a soft swelling at the point of the elbow. Pain is minimal or absent, except when pressure is applied to the swollen bursa, but sometimes there can be considerable discomfort. Local treatment with ice for the first 8 hours followed by heat with compression dressings is usually the only therapy needed. Differential diagnosis requires ruling out local infection or olecranon bursitis as manifestations of rheumatoid arthritis or crystalline synovitis (gout or pseudogout). Infection is suggested when there is marked tenderness, heat or redness, or desquamation of the overlying skin, and fever. Leukocytosis is too infrequent to be helpful in suggesting infection. Operationally, when the inflammation is prominent, the bursa must be aspirated and cultured, and the fluid must be inspected for crystals. Rheumatoid arthritis is suggested by involvement of other joints; crystalline synovitis at the elbow is suggested by objective synovitis with an abrupt onset of pain without a history of trauma and pain at rest. It looks like infection and an aspiration for diagnosis is mandatory.

Epicondylitis

Epicondylitis is the most common cause of pain in the elbow. Despite a literature that starts in the late 1800s, there is still disagreement about its etiology, natural history, and optimal treatment. The entity is also known as tennis elbow, radiohumeral bursitis (synovitis), tendinitis of the common extensor origin, traumatic epicondylitis, periostitis (lateral epicondyle), epicondylalgia externa, and epicondylitis humeri. The symptoms have been attributed to low-grade infection, aseptic necrosis, neuritis of the branches of the radial nerve or of the dorsal antebrachial cutaneous nerve, irritation of the collateral ligament, irritation of the orbiculary ligament, or microscopic tears of the common tendons of the finger extensors, etc. — a total of 26 putative causes — all of which attest to our ignorance about this common condition.

Tennis elbow occurs in patients who repeatedly pronate and supinate the arm with their wrist extended. A similar syndrome occurs at the medial epicondyle. Seen in world class as well as amateur tennis players, it frequently occurs in sedentary occupations where no clear-cut antecedent stresses can be identified. Four syndromes are recognized:

1. An acute course following indirect trauma where disability dates from the acute pain and a "feeling" of something giving way at the elbow during a strenuous act. On the other side of the forearm, just below the epicondyle, a swelling appears that subsides in a week or less. Treatment is usually not necessary.

2. A subacute variety following indirect trauma found in younger patients. The onset is gradual and follows vigorous exercise with the arm. The symptoms subside when the elbow is rested, but reappear with more intensity when the activity is resumed, until finally the patient can hardly turn a door handle or lift an object. The syndrome may take a few days or weeks to reach its peak and spontaneous resolution is the rule.

3. With chronic occupational stresses, painful elbow develops insidiously over 1 to 2 months. An injury history is usually not obtainable, but the patient's occupation provides the clue. Although the pain and disability are not so severe as in the acute variety, a spontaneous cure is less common than in the acute type.

4. An acute form following overuse associated with intense pain, night pain and occasional low grade five of less than 101°F. The forearm may be swollen and red but the exam shows normal elbow motion, no synovitis and exquisite tenderness over the epicondyle. A crystalline tenosynovitis is the presumed cause as micro-calcitreations come and go with the symptoms. Infection needs to be excluded.

The examination is virtually diagnostic (Figure 2–3). X-rays are of little value. In one study, 98 consecutive patients with elbow pain were x-rayed. Only 6 of the 98 had any radiological findings at all. These findings consisted of calcium deposits in the soft tissues and were of questionable clinical significance, since the x-ray results did not alter the treatment or the outcome.

The literature on treatment of epicondylitis suggests that all therapies work or nothing works. Although the criteria for diagnosis are generally uniform, no studies have controls. In all studies, the elbow is rested, the most important therapeutic maneuver. The principal outcome, pain relief, is difficult to quantitate.

Enthusiasts exist for manipulation, immobilization of the elbow in extension, short-wave diathermy, local infrared, ultraviolet, x-ray, ultrasound, faradic stimulation, cauterization, painting with iodine, strapping, massage, and injection intraarticularly or over the point of maximal tenderness with agents from carbolic acid to steroids and procainamide. Surgical approaches include division of the common extensor tendon origin, excision of the tender area, resection of the obicular ligament, z-shaped tenotomy to lengthen the tendon, removal of the radiohumeral bursa, etc.

We recommend conservative measures. Immobilization and the application of ice should be initiated during the acute phase; heat might be applied later on, and antiinflammatory analgesic agents should be administered, along with advice

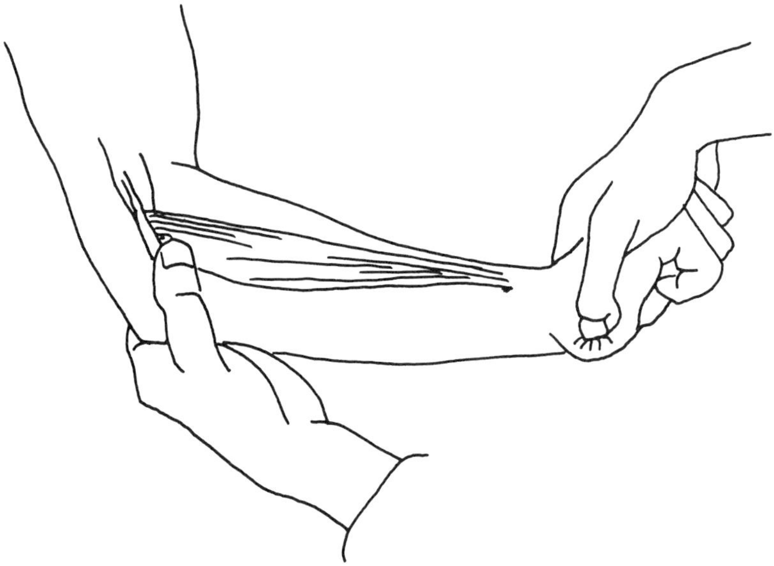

Figure 2–3. Tests for tennis elbow. With lateral epicondylitis (tennis elbow), the pain is reproduced by resisting the examiner's attempt at forcing flexion of the wrist or by pressure over the epicondyle.

about avoiding stressful activities. In resting the elbow, the position of optimal function is approximately 70° to 80° of flexion with the forearm in slight supination. Improvement should occur during the next 1 to 3 weeks. If there is no improvement, radiological examination is indicated to look for an avulsion fracture. A firm forearm band an inch or two distal to the epicondyle or a splint to keep the wrist in a neutral position to reduce tension on the tendinous insertion are useful measures to prevent or treat epicondylitis. Failing this, injection of corticosteroids may be tried, although there are no adequate clinical trials, at the site of maximal tenderness if the x-ray is negative and symptoms persist. For the acute inflammatory tenosynovitis variety, the fourth subset, described above, an antiinflammatory such as indomethacin, is useful.

Pulled Elbow

A pulled elbow results from the head of the radius being pulled partially through the annular ligament. Children are predisposed because the radial head is small in relation to the annular ligament or because in certain positions of the arm — especially when the arm is pronated — the shape of the head may make it liable to be pulled out of place. Fibers to the annular ligament may actually tear in some children.

Though pulled elbow is common and well recognized by orthopedists, it is often unrecognized by primary care physicians, even those dealing with many children. It presents in children less than 6 years old as an acute onset of elbow pain and inability to use one arm. There is slightly limited supination of the forearm but no swelling of the elbow and no loss of elbow flexion. Radiographs are of little use in this diagnosis. The treatment is a simple manipulation performed without anesthesia, holding the lower part of the humerus firmly, and with the thumb over the head of the radius, flicking the forearm into full supination.

PAIN OF THE WRIST

Pain of the wrist may result from strain, fracture of the navicular bone, osteoarthritis of the first carpal metacarpal joint, cervical radiculopathy, radiation of pain from the shoulder or elbow, carpal tunnel syndrome, or DeQuervain's disease (tendinitis). In the initial sorting of complaints of wrist pain, one should not miss navicular fracture, crystalline synovitis, or infectious arthritis (gonococcal tenosynovitis). The wrist is the classic site for both pseudogout and gonococcal tenosynovitis.

Fracture of the Navicular Bone, Other Trauma

Fracture of the navicular bone is suspected with a history of trauma and tenderness in the anatomical snuff box. An x-ray at the time of the injury may confirm the diagnosis. If the x-ray is negative initially, a repeat film 2 weeks later may show a healing fracture line. Early recognition of a navicular fracture is important so that treatment (cast or rigid splint) may be applied to prevent aseptic necrosis of the bone. Ligamentous tears can sometime be detected only by an arthrogram with stress views.

Osteoarthritis (OA) of the First Carpometacarpal Joint (CMC)

The carpometacarpal joint is the second most common joint involved with osteoarthritis. Patients complain of wrist pain aggravated by sustained grip. On examination, the wrist is normal but the base of the thumb feels crepitant when the thumb is rotated. The area of tenderness on motion is medial to the anatomical snuff box and should not be confused with fracture, dislocation, DeQuervain's disease, or aseptic necrosis of the navicular carpal. X-ray detail of the area merely confirms the diagnosis.

As with osteoarthritis of other joints, the treatment is reassurance, patient education, and joint rest. After a flare up of symptoms, the pain gets better within 1 to 2 weeks. For someone who needs to use the hands or who has repeated episodes, the joint may be immobilized with a thumb splint.

Carpal Tunnel Syndrome

The carpal tunnel syndrome results from compression of the median nerve as it passes under the volar carpal ligament. It is associated with repetitive trauma,

TABLE 2–6. CAUSES OF CARPAL TUNNEL SYNDROME

Idiopathic (majority)
Trauma
Repetitive trauma
Reduced space in carpal tunnel
Tenosynovitis
Inflammatory arthritis
Acromegaly
Pregnancy (especially third trimester)
Hypothyroidism
Chronic renal failure/hemodialysis
Amyloid
S/p fracture
Increased susceptibility to pressure
Diabetes mellitus
Other polyneuropathies

previous fracture, obesity, pregnancy, rheumatoid arthritis, hypothroidism, and amyloidosis. For all practical purposes, an etiologic diagnosis does not change the management (Table 2–6). The classic case presents as numbness and tingling radiating from the wrist to the palmar surface of the thumb, index, and radial half of the ring finger, frequently with nighttime awakening or forearm symptoms. Thenar atrophy occurs in advanced cases. The classic physical findings are not so specific nor so sensitive compared to nerve conduction testing, which is the only way to diagnose the condition absolutely. A positive Tinel's sign elicited by percussing the median nerve at the volar surface of the wrist reproduces the pain and paresthesia in the distribution of the nerve. Phalen and reverse Phalen maneuvers (hyperextension and flexion, respectively, of the wrist for 1 minute) can also be used to reproduce the symptoms. Strength testing shows diminished power to oppose the thumb and index finger. Nerve conduction studies show some denervation after symptoms have been present for 8 weeks and a decrement in nerve conduction velocity of the median nerve across the wrist.

Electrophysiologic studies are valuable to exclude other sources of median nerve compression in the forearm or cervical root compression (so-called double crush syndrome).

Compression of the median nerve and its branches by hypertrophied or otherwise swollen muscles in the forearm can appear to be carpal tunnel syndrome. The symptoms include "pseudo carpal tunnel" (sublimis) syndrome, interosseous nerve syndrome, and pronator teres syndrome. Muscles supplied by these branches can be examined specifically by nerve conduction studies. The lack of response to the wrist splinting or exacerbation of the symptoms by resisted pronation or supination of the forearm are clues that other forearm compression syndromes may be present.

Other important nerve-root compressions occurring in the upper extremities include ulnar neuropathy at the elbow, usually traumatic, and "Saturday night palsy," or radial nerve compression at the axilla due to crutches or to falling asleep in an awkward position with the arm over a chair. These two syndromes can be readily identified on physical examination by the distribution of weakness. Ulnar neuropathy should produce some weakness of abduction of the little finger, whereas radial neuropathy produces weakness of the ability to hold the thumb in the "hitchhiking" position against resistance.

Surgical decompression or carpal tunnel release, is indicated if there is no clear and significant improvement in symptoms or if there is weakness or atrophy of the intrinsic muscles of the hand. Nerve conduction tests of the median nerve confirm the diagnosis in atypical cases and document clinical progression or improvement, but are generally not needed if surgery has been already decided upon. If there is no weakness or atrophy of the intrinsic muscles of the hand, conservative management of splinting and/or local corticosteroids into the tunnel and treatment of the underlying conditions may be tried and the patient should be followed for the next 2 to 4 weeks. By that time, improvement should occur. "A little improvement" should warrant another attempt at conservative management. Worsening pains or evidence of neuromyopathy is an indication to refer the patient.

DeQuervain's Disease

DeQuervain's disease is a tenosynovitis of the conjoined tendons of the long abductor and short extensor of the thumb across the radial styloid at the wrist. Tenosynovitis of other tendons crossing the wrist dorsally, a condition not to be confused with DeQuervain's disease, is a common presentation of disseminated gonococcal disease. The most common cause of DeQuervain's disease is trauma. Tenderness at the radial styloid in the anatomical snuff box may be present. The diagnosis is confirmed by flexing the thumb into the palm with the other fingers flexed over the thumb and bending the wrist in an ulnar direction at the wrist (Finkelstein's test), which reproduces sharp pain. In addition, local signs such as swelling of the tendon sheath, crepitus, or a rub may be recognized. In this condition, splinting of the wrist in a position of function, slightly dorsiflexed, is useful, and improvement usually ensues within 2 or 3 weeks. Steroid injections into the tendon sheath are helpful for refractory cases but should be referred if the physician is not experienced.

FINGER PAIN

Aside from trauma, pain or stiffness in the fingers is commonly due to osteoarthritis of the fingers or to flexor tenosynovitis.

In sorting out hand pain, one should not miss:

1. Neurovascular compromise (median, ulnar, nerve compression, occlusive vascular disease)
2. Tendon rupture, dislocation.
3. Infection (felon, paronychia, pyogenic tenosynovitis, cellulitis)
4. Hypertrophic pulmonary osteoarthropathy

"Trigger finger or snapping finger" results from interference of the normal movement of finger tendon through the sheaths. Passive flexion and extension of the fingers are normal, but active flexion and extension result in locking and discomfort. A nodule in the flexor tendon or swelling and crepitation of the tendon sheath may be appreciated. Flexor tenosynovitis may be treated conservatively with splinting. Whenever this fails, a corticosteroid injection into the involved area generally works. When conservative management is exhausted, a surgical release is usually curative.

The most common arthritis of the hands is osteoarthritis, recognized on inspection as Heberden's nodes (distal interphalangeal joint) and/or Bouchard's nodes (proximal interphlalangeal joint). It occurs commonly as a symmetrical process in older women. When nodes are confined to one finger or to one hand, they are usually the result of significant injury or avulsion of the extensor tendon. The first carpometacarpal joint may be involved with degenerative changes between the trapezium and anatomical snuff box. X-rays are unnecessary for diagnosis, management, or following the patient.

Herberden's nodes, unassociated with osteoarthritis of the knees or hips, develops primarily in women without symptoms or with only minor aching over several years. Occasionally developing Heberden's nodes go through an acute stage resembling a paronychia. In addition, in both Heberden's and Bouchard's nodes, a small cystic structure containing hyaluronic acid with or without protein may form over the dorsum of this joint (mucinous cyst). When the osteoarthritic nodes are fully developed, a flexion deformity or deviation to one side are common. As a rule, osteoarthritis of the fingers cause little disability, except during the earlier stages, when deep aching pain follows finger use and is aggravated by cooling. Persons with first carpometacarpal involvement complain of pain increased by gripping or twisting hand motion. Periodic flares are usually precipitated by heavy finger use and resolve with complete joint rest over a few days or over weeks to months if the fingers are continually traumatized. With progression of the condition, symptoms diminish as finger movement is restricted by the nodes themselves.

Persons with mild joint complaints due to osteoarthritis of the fingers are "treated" by explaining what the condition is and what it is not. Patients want to know what to expect, which is that the condition will not progress or "spread," and that it is not an inflammatory arthritis such as rheumatoid arthritis, with all its bad associations.

Activities that produce pain should be avoided, but that is not always possible nor practical. Where it is not, splinting of particularly bothersome joints is extremely effective treatment. Spandex gloves worn at night help many patients and is worth a trial. In a patient with bilateral involvement, using a glove on the dominant hand (which is usually the most symptomatic side) can be compared with the other side. Let the patient provide his or her own control in this way. Surgery for osteoarthritis of the fingers is justified rarely and only to improve function.

REFERENCES

Basmajian JV: Reflex cervical muscle spasm: Treatment by diazepam, phenobarbital or placebo. Arch Phys Med Rehab 64:121–124, 1983.

Belsole RJ: DeQuervain's tenosynovitis diagnostic and operative complications. Orthopedics 4:899–903, 1981.

Binder A, Hazelman BL, Parr G, Roberts S: A controlled study of oral prednisolone in frozen shoulder. Br J Rheum 25:288–292, 1986.

Binder A, Parr G, Hazelman B: Ultrasound in tennis elbow. Ann Rheum Dis 42:309–312, 1983.

Binder AI, Bulgen DY, Hazelman BL, Roberts S: Frozen shoulder: A long-term prospective study. Ann Rheum Dis 43:361–364, 1984.

Bizk TE, Pinals RS: Frozen shoulder. Semin Arthitis Rheum 11:440–442, 1982.

Bland JH: *Disorders of the Cervical Spine: Diagnosis and Medical Management.* WB Saunders, Philadelphia, 1987.

Bulgen DY, Binder AI, Hazelman BL, Dutton J, Roberts S: Frozen shoulder: Prospective clinical study with an evaluation of three treatment regimens. Ann Rheum Dis 43:353–360, 1984.

Dorwat BB: Carpal tunnel syndrome: A review. Semin Arthitis Rheum 14:134–140, 1984.

Downing D, Weinstein A: Ultrasound therapy of subacromial bursitis: A double blind trial. Arthritis Rheum 26:37–, 1983.

Green SM: Tenosynovitis of the hand. Orthop Rev 6:55–64, 1985.

Ho G Jr, Mickolich DJ: Bacterial infection of the superficial subcutaneous bursae. Clin Rheum Dis 12:437–457, 1986.

Hollingworth GR, Ellis RM, Hattersley TM: Comparison of injection techniques for shoulder pain: Results of a double blind, randomized study. Br Med J 287:1339–1341, 1983.

Howard FM: Controversies in nerve entrapment syndromes in the forearm and wrist. Orthop Clin North Am 17:375–281, 1986.

Illingworth CM: Pulled elbow: A study of 100 patients. Br Med J 2:672–674, 1975.

Kelsey JL, Githens PB, Walter SD, et al.: An epidemiological study of acute prolapsed cervical intervertebral disc. J Bone Joint Surg [Am] 66A:907–914, 1984.

Matsen FA, Kirby RM: Office evaluation and management of shoulder pain. Orthop Clin North Am 13:453–475, 1982.

Nakamo KK: Neck pain. In Kelley WN, Harris ED Jr, Ruddy S, et al. (eds). *Textbook of Rheumtology*. 3rd edition. WB Saunders, Philadelphia, 1989, pp. 471–490.

Neer CS, Craig EV, Fukuda H. Cuff-tear arthropathy. *J Bone Joint Surg* [Am] 65A:1232–1244, 1983.

Neviaser RJ, Neviaser TJ: The frozen shoulder: Diagnosis and treatment. Clin Orthop 223:59–63, 1987.

Petri M, Dobrow R, Neiman R, Whiting-O'Keefe Q, Seaman WE: Randomized, double blind placebo-controlled study of the treatment of the painful shoulder. Arthritis Rheum 30:1040–1045, 1987.

Phalen GS: The carpal-tunnel syndrome: Seventeen years' experience in diagnosis and treatment of six hundred fifty-four hands. J Bone Joint Surg [Am] 48:211–228, 1966.

Schutzer SF, Gossling HR: The treatment of reflex sympathetic dystrophy syndrome. J Bone Joint Surg [Am] 66A:625–629, 1984.

Subbarao J, Stillwell GK: Reflex sympathetic dystrophy syndrome of the upper extremity: Analysis of total outcome of management of 125 cases. Arch Phys Med Rehabil 62:549–552, 1981.

Thomas D, Williams RA, Smith DS: The frozen shoulder: A review of manipulative treatment. Rheum Rehabil 19:173–179, 1980.

White RH, Paull DM, Fleming KW: Rotator cuff tendinitis: Comparison of subacromial injection of a long-acting corticosteroid versus oral indomethacin therapy. J Rheumatol 13:608–613, 1986.

Yu YL, Woo E, Huang CY: Cervical spondylitic myelopathy and radiculopathy. Acta Neurol Scand 75:367–373, 1987.

Zylbergold RS, Piper MC: Cervical spine disorders. A comparison of three types of traction. Spine 10:867–871, 1985.

3

Pain in the Lower Extremity

Other than visits for traumatic conditions, the majority of visits to the office for musculoskeletal complaints are for low back pain, neck pain, shoulder pain, and a variety of nonarticular rheumatic syndromes. Inflammatory arthritis is uncommon. The most chronic "arthritis" is osteoarthritis, which is more properly viewed as a primary disorder of cartilage with secondary structural changes; synovitis plays only a minor part in the pathogenesis of the disorder. The most common chronic inflammatory arthritis is rheumatoid arthritis, and it represents less than 1% of all office visits. The chapters on musculoskeletal complaints reflect this epidemiology. This chapter discusses, specifically, hip, knee, and foot pain.

KNEE PAIN

In an ambulatory setting, knee pain is due to strains and sprains, bursitis, chondromalacia patellae, and osteoarthritis in descending order of frequency. In children, Osgood–Schlatter disease and osteochondritis dessicans would rank before chondromalacia patellae, and osteoarthritis would almost never be seen. In both children and adults, inflammatory or infectious arthritis is uncommon but must be recognized early.

Diagnostic Strategy

The three major syndromes of knee pain are (Table 3–1):

1. Knee pain with joint effusion, with or without instability
2. Knee pain without joint effusion
3. Knee pain with or without effusion and with locking or giving way

In knee pain with joint effusion (intraarticular conditions), inflammatory conditions such as infections, inflammatory arthropathy (juvenile or adult

TABLE 3–1. KNEE PAIN SYNDROMES

Knee Pain With Effusion

Inflammatory arthritis
Infection
Internal derangement, chronic
Bleed
Baker's cyst
Misc
  Hypertrophic pulmonary osteoarthropathy
  Relapsing polychondritis
  Intermittent hydrarthrosis
  Etc.

Knee Pain Without Effusion

Bursitis
Tendonitis
Osteoarthritis
Chondromalacia patellae
Referred (trochanteric bursitis, slipped femoral capital epiphysis, osteoarthritis of hip, Paget's, etc.)
Osseous lesion
  Paget's
  Hypertrophic pulmonary osteoarthropathy
  Avascular necrosis
  Larsen–Johansson — osteochondritis of patellar poles
  Tumor (osteochondroma, giant cyst, osteogenic sarcoma, etc.)

Knee Pain With or Without Effusion *and* With Locking

Internal derangement
Loose body (tumor, cartilage fragment)
Lateral discoid meniscus (in younger patients)
Recurrent subluxation of patella

rheumatoid arthritis, gout, pseudogout, Reiter's disease, other spondyloarthropathies, etc.) should be considered and can often be ruled out by tapping the joint and finding joint fluid with a low cell count (fewer than 1000 white blood cells), no crystals, and negative gram stain and culture. Sprains (i.e., rupture), strains (stretching of a ligament), and meniscus injuries may also present with a small effusion.

In knee pain without joint effusion (extraarticular conditions), bone tumor, chondromalacia patellae, osteochondritis dessicans, osteoarthritis, and referred pain from the hip (slipped femoral capital epiphysis, osteoarthritis of the hip, etc.) are possibilities. Acute sprains, strains, and meniscal injuries may also occur without joint effusion.

When there is knee pain with locking or giving way, one must think of a discoid lateral meniscus in children up to 8 years of age, dislocation of the patellae, meniscal injuries, loose bodies, and a lax knee secondary to an unstable knee or quadriceps atrophy.

Knee Examination

A careful history and examination to recognize synovitis and to localize the pain further by reproducing the pain during the examination are all that are needed for proper diagnosis in the majority of cases. If symptoms persist beyond 2 weeks or the examination is *completely* normal, or if the pain is persistent and unrelated to activity, think of a lesion of bone or referred pain.

The patient should be observed in a standing position for valgus or varus deformities. Knee pain secondary to genu valgum or a pronated foot arise from the attachment of the medial collateral ligament. Palpate the anatomical structures systematically to identify discrete painful regions. The clinically important bursa of the knee are the prepatellar bursa, superficial and deep infrapatellar bursa, and the pes anserine bursa (Figure 3–1). The insertion of the infrapatellar tendon and the biceps femoris tendon are frequently involved in injuries. In meniscus injury, tenderness is maximal below the medial femoral condyle and accurately predicts the site of a tear found at surgery. Large effusions are evident upon inspection and are confirmed by ballotting the patella with the leg extended to feel the characteristic sponginess. A small-to-moderate effusion is suggested by the bulge sign, which is done by milking the fluid into the suprapatellar pouch and then stroking the joint space on one side to elicit a wave on the other. Since an effusion points to an intraarticular source of symptoms, and the distinction between intraarticular and extraarticular diseases is central to diagnosis (Figure 1–2), eliciting these physical signs is key to sorting out knee complaints.

Crepitus with joint movement is felt over the joint line and may be appreciated as being close to the hand and "coarse," in which case chondromalacia patellae or degenerative arthritis is likely. "Fine" crepitus is appreciated in inflammatory arthritis.

Joint stability is checked by stressing, in turn, the medial and lateral collateral ligaments and the anterior and posterior cruciate ligaments. Since the medial collateral ligament is critical to stability, an isolated tear will lead to joint instability; whereas, a similar defect in the lateral collateral ligament may not be as significant. Most ligamentous injuries occur on the medial side.

To test the medial collateral ligament, the patient's knee should be flexed slightly to eliminate the stabilizing contribution of the cruciates, and valgus stress is applied in an attempt to open the knee joint on the medial side. A defect may be palpated. Relieving stress on the injured joint may produce a "clunk" as the tibia and femur close sharply. The lateral collateral ligament is tested in a similar fashion by varus stress.

The cruciate ligaments are checked by the anterior and posterior drawer sign. For this test, the patient is supine on the examining table with the head down. If a patient tries to see what the examiner is doing, hamstring tightening may occur. The hip is flexed to 45° and the knee to 80° to 90° degrees, and the foot is placed on the table top. The examiner's hands are placed about the upper part of the tibia, with the forefingers palpating the hamstrings to ensure that they are relaxed. Then gently and repeatedly pull and push the proximal part of the leg to and fro. The test should be done first with the foot and leg externally rotated beyond the neutral position, then internally rotated as much as is comfortably possible, and finally in the neutral position. The injured extremity should be compared with the uninjured extremity.

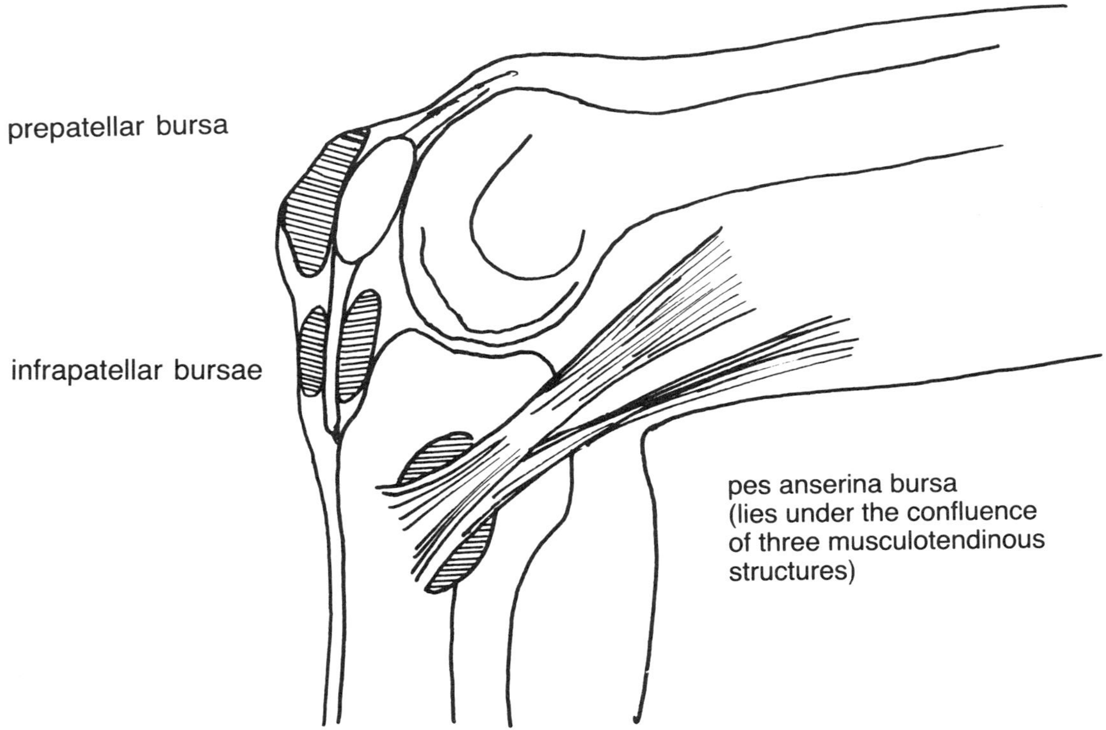

Figure 3–1. The clinically important bursae of the knee viewed from the medial aspect.

The push portion of the drawer test is used to demonstrate the presence or absence of a posterior drawer sign. If the posterior drawer sign is positive, the tibial tuberosity can be seen displaced posteriorly on the affected side compared with the normal side. Swelling of the affected knee, either intraarticular or periarticular, can produce the illusion of posterior displacement when there is none.

Finally, quadriceps strength should be quantitated. A simple grading scheme amenable to serial observations is the patient's ability to resist the examiner's outstretched fingers (four fingers resisted down to one finger resisted).

Initial Conservative Treatment of Knee Pain

The treatment options for acute and subacute knee pain are similar. Common to treatment of all of the conditions to be discussed is joint rest, prevention of muscle atrophy, and, to a much lesser extent, analgesics (see Chapter 5). More specific interventions will be noted where relevant. Joint rest is accomplished by non-weight bearing, bed rest, or the use of appliances.

Appliances, such as canes or crutches, are indicated when joint pain, destruction, or muscle weakness will not allow the lower extremities to tolerate the normal stresses of weight bearing without pain or when non-weight bearing is desired to accelerate healing. A cane should always be fitted with the largest rubber tip for maximum traction and safety. When crutches are not indicated, but optimal stability is desired, a crab cane which provides three points of contact with the ground, or a quadruple cane, which provides four points of contact, may be employed. Adequate elbow flexion and upper extremity strength is necessary for optimal support and elevation while a person is ambulating with a cane. A properly fitted cane will have its highest point level with the person's greater trochanter. When a person is standing erect, the feet and the cane tip should form a stable base, with the tip placed about 8″ ahead of and lateral to the toes of the unaffected extremity. The shoulders should not be hunched up; the elbows should be flexed about 20° while the cane is being used for balance. If the patient bends forward, the cane is too short. A person should hold the cane in the hand opposite the involved hip or knee.

The most easily obtainable crutch is the axillary type. Correct crutch measurement is essential for proper crutch walking patterns and for preventing excessive stress on the upper extremities. Many formulas exist for fitting crutches, but, ultimately, adjustments are made on the basis of comfort and minimizing arm fatigue after crutch use.

Axillary crutches that are too long limit the patient's ability to manipulate them and may cause brachial plexus injury. When crutches are too short, the patient leans forward and stresses the back. Before a person is measured for an axillary crutch, it should be dressed with a rubber tip and hand cushions. Measurements for the total crutch length are taken from 2″ below the anterior axillary fold to a point on the floor 4″ to 6″ anterior and lateral to the shoes. When the crutches are held at this point on the floor, the patient is in the tripod position, which is the initial stance for all gait patterns. The handpiece on axillary crutches should allow about 30° of elbow flexion with the patient's wrist in dorsiflexion. Elbow flexion is necessary to provide adequate leverage to lift the body when the person bears down on the handpiece. If a person needs crutches for any length of time, he or she should learn different crutch gait patterns to prevent fatigue of one set of muscles.

Appliances such as canes, crutches, or splints are occasionally resisted because of the association with being crippled and/or infirm, even though they are of considerable benefit in reducing the mechanical stresses on a joint. (Margaret Mead preferred a staff to a cane.) When prescribing an appliance, emphasize that it need not be permanent.

The importance of identifying activities that stress the involved joints cannot be overemphasized. Minor adjustments in routine, job, or posture can make a tremendous difference. The patient with cervical degenerative joint disease should avoid bifocals. Patients have been "cured" of joint symptoms in their fingers by stopping their knitting. The question, "What makes your joint pain worse?" helps to identify stressful activities.

Applications of heat or cold may provide symptomatic relief without resorting to medications. Though there are different opinions about the usefulness of these measures, the following statements hold:

1. There is no proven advantage of deep heat (diathermy) over superficial heat.
2. There is no advantage of superficial heat (moist hot packs, hot packs, hot soaks, paraffin, hot mud, and hot sand) over superficial cold applications.
3. There are individual preferences for cold versus warm applications, and the desirable therapy must be arrived at empirically.
4. In general, the more acute the process, the more likely cold applications will help; the more subacute the process, the more likely warm, and particularly moist-warm, applications will be of benefit.
5. Superficial heat is contraindicated in the presence of neuropathy and impaired circulation, due to the likelihood of an inadvertent burn.

Towels soaked in hot water, soaks, and hot baths are effective ways to apply moist heat to large areas. Stretch gloves applied at bedtime or hot soaks can be used for the hands. Electric heating pads commonly cause accidental burns, particularly when patients fall asleep during the treatment. If moist heat is to be used for any length of time, hydroculator packs may be used. These packs, containing a silica gel, maintain moist heat for up to 45 minutes.

Maintaining muscle strength is particularly important for painful conditions of the knee. Even an athlete will show quadriceps wasting after several days with the leg immobilized. Good quadriceps strength helps maintain knee stability. "Quad setting," is done with the leg extended and slightly externally rotated to utilize the vasas medialis. Motion is judged by observing the upward motion of the patella and contraction of the quadriceps muscle. The contraction is sustained for 8 seconds, then relaxed. This exercise is performed 15 to 30 times a day. Wasted muscles fade from the patients' body image: they may have to be reminded what active contraction feels like by feeling the contracted muscle

TABLE 3–2. KNEE PAIN — DON'T MISS

Acute torn ligament
Infection
Referred pain (hip, back)
Anterior compartment syndrome
Peroneal palsy
Fracture
Hemarthrosis

bulk while exercising. As muscle power improves, exercises against gradually increasing resistance are introduced.

Heavy resistance exercises with low repetition develops power. Low resistance with frequent repetition develops endurance. Isometric exercises are used when joint motion needs to be avoided or is not possible. Resistive exercises are rhythmic dynamic exercises for development of strength. They use maximal resistance and are increased gradually until strength improves.

In summary, the key to diagnosing and managing knee pain is the history and specific anatomical localization by examination. In the initial office visit, one should be looking for ligamentous laxity, quadriceps strength, synovitis, and discrete areas of maximal tenderness. Do not miss the conditions that cause knee pain in Table 3–2. For all other causes, joint rest and the preservation of muscle strength are the cornerstones of management. The following sections will detail the major knee pain syndromes and specific therapies.

KNEE PAIN WITHOUT JOINT EFFUSION

Sprains of the Knee, Running Injuries

Sprains vary from mild, with minimal stretching or tearing of fibers without loss of integrity of the ligament, to a complete tear of the ligament with or without avulsion of the bone to which it is attached. In mild sprains, full recovery is expected with conservative treatment; in severe sprains or tears of the knee, early surgery is essential.

Chronic strain of the knee, almost always on the medial aspect, occurs in persons with genu valgus and persons with pronated feet. The latter is a common problem of joggers and distance runners who repeatedly traumatize the medial ligaments and tendons with running. Treatment is simple — an insert or support (for example, Dr. Scholl's arch support or a shoe with a varus wedge) or a specially fitted orthoses. For the person with genu valgus and a healthy medial compartment who has medial knee pain, a similar "plastic osteotomy" can be extremely effective in mechanical stresses.

Running on banked roads may also cause ligament strain. A normal foot may be forced into pronation, causing medial knee pain, or supination, inducing lateral knee pain. The treatment here is not in shoe manipulation, but in running on flat roads.

Bursitis and Tendinitis Lesions of the Knee

Although bursa may occur wherever tendon join bony surfaces or muscles ride over muscles, the clinically important bursa of the knee are the pes anserine, infrapatellar, prepatellar, and suprapatellar bursae (Figure 3–1). Inflammation of the bursa or tendons may occur as an isolated event or with inflammatory arthritis or other primary knee problems.

The diagnosis is made by careful examination of the knee to identify a discrete area of pain and tenderness at an anatomical site of a bursa or tendon insertion. The knee joint itself should have no fluid and a normal range of motion if bursitis or tendinitis is the sole cause of pain. Other signs of inflammation such as heat and swelling may not be as obvious. Tendinitis may have an associated and occasionally audible rub with movement of the tendon. Discrete swelling is uncommon and tenderness tends to be "linear" following a distribution of a tendon. Bursitis and tendinitis frequently occur together, and clinical differentiation may be difficult. The treatment, however, is the same. Pain that is severe enough to interfere with sleep is due to severe structural damage of the joint, irritation or damage to the nerve, or inflammation of a bursa or tendon sheath. Of those three possibilities bursitis (or tendinitis) is the most common of nocturnal pain.

Painless swelling of bursa is frequent and causes symptoms by being vulnerable to minor trauma. Prepatellar bursitis, housemaid's knees, or nun's knees are commonly painless and result from kneeling on hard surfaces. The treatment of bursitis is as follows: For bursa swelling without clinical evidence of inflammation, complete aspiration of the swelling is followed by applying a pressure dressing for a week and protecting the area from trauma by either a pad or avoiding kneeling. Recurrences are treated in the same manner. For an inflamed bursa, complete aspiration and a local injection with Xylocaine® (1 to 2 ml of Xylocaine 1%) and/or corticosteroids (10 mg of methylprednisone) is effective. No formal clinical trials have compared this with oral drug therapy, local heat, or local cold, but the clinician's lore suggests treatment with injection therapy is the most effective.

Osteoarthritis (OA) of the Knee

Osteoarthritis is the most common arthritic condition of the knee and may involve each of the three distinct articular surfaces: the patello-femoral, lateral, and medial compartments. It is the major cause of disabling knee pain in elderly, middle-aged, and obese persons. In its earliest stages, pain occurs with walking and increases as walking is continued. In contrast to the pain from arterial insufficiency, which usually appears at a relatively constant distance, pain from osteoarthritis occurs at different distances walked before the onset of pain. In addition, the pain of osteoarthritis persists longer than the few minutes generally required to relieve ischemic pain.

In advanced disease, the joint is consistently painful on weight bearing, with periodic acute exacerbation and pain at rest. Flares may result from ligamentous strains, associated bursitis, and traumatic or rarely crystalline (hydroxyapatite or calcium pyrophosphate crystals) synovitis. Rupture of a popliteal cyst may rarely cause an exacerbation. The event is less traumatic than in ruptured Baker's cysts associated with rheumatoid arthritis because of the lower content of enzymes in the fluid of osteoarthrosis. With advanced disease, the cartilage is worn through and bone grates on bone with each movement of the joint. Pain with each step of weight bearing, at rest, and at night are the features of an end-stage (or nearly end-stage) joint. The knee is frequently unstable as well. Medical management is symptomatic.

On examination, bony enlargement, deformity, pain, and/or crepitus on motion without evidence of synovitis are the key features of osteoarthritis. X-ray examination done standing shows the features of osteoarthritis: unequal joint space narrowing, eburnation, osteophytes, and subchondral bone cysts.

Osteoarthritis rarely passes undiagnosed. It is usually only in the very early stages of primary osteoarthritis when there may be symptoms with little clinical or radiological abnormality that there is any difficulty in recognizing it. The diagnosis in such early cases may be suspected after the exclusion of other conditions, but a definite diagnosis requires a period of observation. In practice, the most common difficulty is being certain that osteoarthritis confirmed by x-ray examination is responsible for the symptoms.

The exact pathophysiology of osteoarthritis is unknown. At least one factor is the articular cartilage itself. With increasing age, some degree of degenerative change in articular cartilage is universal, but the age of appearance of the changes, their rate of progression, and the severity vary greatly. The amount of joint use seems to be a major determinant of the severity of the osteoarthritic changes. If a joint is subjected to excessive stresses by virtue of trauma, obesity, prior inflammation, or malformation, changes appear prematurely and progress more rapidly. If joint movement is restricted, osteoarthritic changes are arrested; osteoarthritic changes in a paralyzed limb of a patient who becomes hemiplegic are arrested, while in the normal limb osteoarthritis changes steadily increase in extent and severity.

The prognosis of the average patient with osteoarthritis of the knee or hip depends on the age of onset and on whether the process is primary or secondary. Asymmetrical involvement is likely to progress. The variation is quite striking. The younger the age of onset, the more likely the progression. Secondary causes of osteoarthritis add to the natural process and are usually associated with more severe disease.

Treatment of osteoarthritis of the knee

The goals of conservative medical treatment of osteoarthritis of the knee are:

1. Pain relief by relieving mechanical stresses, joint rest, and medication
2. Maintaining function by preventing quadriceps atrophy and deformity

In theory, salicylates inhibit cathepsin and possibly other enzymes, and also arrest cartilaginous degradation of cartilage. When given early in antiinflammatory dosages, salicylates prevent fibrillation. Once fibrillation occurs, there is evidence that salicylates or any other drug alter the natural course of osteoarthritis.

Short-term clinical trials of various drugs in the treatment of osteoarthritis suggest that most people with osteoarthritis improve regardless of the treatment, and possibly indicate that strong placebo effects exist; that joint rest is the single most important ingredient, or a combination of the above. In one study, 86% of 64 patients with osteoarthritis had symptomatic improvement after weekly subcutaneous injections of saline. In another study, nearly 60% of 182 patients with osteoarthritis had some relief from lactose tablets, and 50% of those who did not respond or who relapsed improved after saline injections.

Medications are used primarily for their analgesic and antiinflammatory properties. Spirin alone is effective, although some evidence suggests that Indocin® may be more effective in the treatment of osteoarthritis of the hip and knee joints.

Mechanical stresses should be removed whenever possible — the two most important being stresses due to obesity and to malalignment.

Being overweight is associated with increased risk of OA of the knee; losing weight may improve the symptoms of early degenerative arthritis and may possibly delay its progression. Losing weight, particularly in the age group principally affected by osteoarthritis is no mean feat, but some patients can be motivated by understanding the condition and the rule of three. The latter says that roughly three times the body weight is transmitted across the knee and that a ten-pound weight loss is equivalent to 30 pounds less across the affected knee. Similarly, a cane, either during periodic exacerbations of symptoms or prolonged use, can reduce the amount of impact across the damaged joint surfaces. Some patients with early disease can literally be "cured" by losing weight or using a cane regularly.

Genu valgum and/or a pronated foot impose additional forces across the medial compartment. Unicompartmental osteoarthritis may be the cause or the effect of this misalignment, but a "rubber osteotomy" (an appropriate shoe insert) in an individual with mild unicompartmental joint space narrowing and genu varus deformity and/or a pronated foot redistributes the forces across the knee and relieves knee pain in a considerable number of individuals. Though not proven, surgical osteotomy in carefully selected patients may delay destruction of the compartment as well.

During acute flare-ups of knee pain, treatable conditions such as bursitis, synovitis, or a ruptured Baker's cyst should not be overlooked. Total or partial rest of the joint, while maintaining the quadriceps mechanism by isometric exercises, reduces pain in 3 days in virtually all patients. Physical modalities are of marginal benefit, but physical therapy has an important role in restoring or maintaining quadriceps strength and in preventing and reducing flexion deformities.

Corticosteroids for osteoarthritis of the knee

Systemic corticosteroids have little value in osteoarthritis. Intraarticular corticosteroids for osteoarthritis appear ineffective or only slightly better than placebo treatment. Miller et al. studied the objective and subjective results of five different types of injections given to 181 patients. The five injections included lactic acid and procaine hydrochloride, procaine hydrochloride alone, saline, hydrocortisone, and a mock injection. They found no difference between the five injections other than that men showed greater subjective improvement than did women, regardless of the injection. A 6-month follow-up showed that patients' conditions were similar to those of the preinjection period.

Repeated intraarticular corticosteroid injections may cause harm. In animals, intraarticular steroids lead to degeneration of the cartilagenous matrix. In rabbits, injection of steroids near the tendon calcaneous led to necrosis of collagen and a decreased inflammatory reaction within several days. These changes showed no evidence of repair after 8 weeks, unlike lesions caused by saline injections near the tendon. These effects seem to be qualitatively worse with repeated injections of steroids. In studies with primates, injections do not appear as harmful. Clinically, there have been scattered reports of enhanced destruction of joints receiving repeated injections of steroids.

If steroids are used for osteoarthritis, care should be taken to avoid injection directly into tendinous and ligamentous structures, to limit the number of injections to no more than six per year and no more than three injections to a single joint, and to avoid vigorous use of the joint after an injection. Never inject when there is any appreciable resistance to the injection.

Surgery for osteoarthritis

The ideal candidate for osteotomy has medial compartment osteoarthritis of the knee, no bone loss, no subluxation, intact ligaments, flexion from 0° to 100+°, and pain with weight bearing.

When pain prevents sleep and occurs with any joint use or requires increasing amounts of analgesics or narcotics, the patient has significant structural damage and medical management is limited.

Total joint replacement, particularly of the hip and knee joints, is extremely successful. For patients who are acceptable surgical risks, have one "worse" joint, are motivated, and are not "too young", surgical results are excellent. In centers where such reconstructive surgery is routine, results for total hip replacements should approach 95% success for pain relief and 80% success for functional improvement. The operative mortality is less than 1%, and the morbidity is less than 1%. The percentages hold true for total knee replacements, except that functional improvement is on the order of 70% and depends on patient motivation.

Total joint replacement is not for patients with unstabilized medical problems who have severe muscle atrophy or whose contractures about the affected joint and, to a lesser extent, who have multiple joint involvement. Likewise, beware of recommending surgery to the poorly motivated patient, or to the patient who is motivated for the wrong reasons. If surgery is seen as a panacea for emotional difficulties at home or at work, or if a patient's life "requires" a disability, a "new" joint may unmask new problems.

Osteochondritis Dissecans

Osteochondritis dissecans is a condition in which a fragment of articular cartilage with subchondral bone has separated from the joint surface. This disorder needs to be differentiated from the common finding of irregular epiphyseal ossification or a separate center of ossification, both of which are variations of the normal condition. In osteochondritis dissecans, the intracondylar portion of the medial femoral condyle is involved in 85% of the cases, and the lateral condyle is involved in 15% of the cases. The fragment may become separated and lie free in the joint (joint mouse) or it may remain in its bed attached by fibrous tissue. The etiology of the lesion is speculative. Convex surfaces of pressure epiphyses are susceptible to avascular necrosis of a segment of subchondral bone, which may become separated from the remaining portions of the epiphyses. The osteocytes die, but the overlying articular cartilage that is nourished by synovial fluid remains alive. An ingrowth of granulated tissue from remaining healthy epiphysis "dissects" between living and dead bone, thereby isolating the necrotic segment.

As the necrotic segment becomes revascularized, bone deposition and bone resorption occur simultaneously and, consequently, the convex surface of the epiphyses may flatten. Providing the overlying articular cartilage remains intact, bone healing eventually takes place. If trauma occurs at this stage, overlying cartilage may tear and the necrotic fragment may become a loose body.

Few or no symptoms or clinical signs occur during the early phase of necrosis; but during the revascularization phase, patients may experience intermittent local pain, usually with weight bearing and after exertion, with relatively little disturbance of joint function. Occasionally, a small joint effusion and atrophy of the quadriceps may be noted. If the necrotic segment becomes detached, however, the symptoms and signs become more marked; should it become completely detached, the patient will complain of intermittent catching or locking of the joint due to the presence of the loose body. The physical findings are scarce and nonspecific.

Many small lesions heal spontaneously over a period of 2 to 3 years without any residual joint incongruity. In general, the onset of symptoms under 13 years of age is associated with complete healing. The onset of symptoms in patients over 13 years is associated with the classical medial lesion, which is prone separate. If the defect is large, degenerative disease of the joint may result over a period of years.

The aims of treatment depend on when the condition is first diagnosed. If the necrotic fragment is not detached, conservative treatment is sufficient. The knee is supported with a bulky dressing, and activity is restricted as required by the symptoms. Temporary relief from weight bearing may encourage healing. Unfortunately, restriction of activity is more easily said than done in the age group that is most afflicted by this condition. If pain becomes severe or there is evidence that the fragment has separated, more drastic therapy is indicated [2], and the patient should be referred to an orthopedic surgeon.

Osgood–Schlatter's Disease (Partial Avulsion of the Tibial Tubercule)

In children, the tibial tubercule is formed by a cartilaginous downward prolongation of the tibial epiphysis. Toward the end of growth, one or more centers of ossification appear in the tibial tubercule and then it becomes most vulnerable to the effects of repeated, forceful traction on the attached patellar tendon. Partial avulsion of the tibial tubercule may rarely lead to avascular necrosis of the avulsed portion, but in most cases this division does not cause a disease. Children between the ages of 10 and 15 years are most frequently affected by subsequent symptoms, however. The onset is insidious and the patient becomes aware of the pain and tenderness over the tibial tubercule; occasionally bilateral involvement is seen. The condition is aggravated by exercise or direct pressure, such as kneeling. Clinically, a prominent subcutaneous swelling is noted at the tibial tubercule. The prominence is tender, and the pain may be reproduced by having the patient extend the knee against resistance. There is no advantage to x-raying the knee when the story and the clinical signs are typical. When symptoms persist with conservative therapy, or the clinical picture is unusual, an x-ray is indicated to look for a bone tumor.

The condition is self-limited, disappearing in nearly all patients when full growth is attained. In such cases, the tubercule ossifies over a period of about 2 years. In an occasional child, the proximal segment fails to unite with the remainder of the tubercule, but remains mobile and persists as a source of local pain and tenderness.

The aim of treatment is to prevent further irritation during the healing phase. This is a difficult task in growing children and consists primarily of avoiding kneeling and jumping; it is not necessary to immobilize the knee nor to restrain the child from running. Rarely, excision of an un-united fragment may be done for pain relief.

CHONDROMALACIA PATELLAE

Knee pain occurring at the patellofemoral joint of individuals, particularly females between ages 16 and 30, is commonly diagnosed as chondromalacia patellae. The term is imprecise and is not based on any generally accepted criteria. The condition is thought to be due to fibrillation of the articular cartilage of the medial patella facet. Generally asymptomatic or transiently symptomatic, these same changes may be identified in "normal" knees beginning at age 20 and universally by age 35. It is not precisely known what causes the knee pain. The cartilage itself has no nerve supply. Although the common symptom is anterior knee pain or retropatella aching, related to quadriceps contraction and forceful extension (going down stairs is more painful than going up stairs), several distinct clinical syndromes are described. In the first, the onset is gradual with pain perceived inside the knee and not sharply localized. Symptoms are provoked by strenuous sports and resolved after 24 to 48 hours. With time, symptoms may occur after minimal effort; and in some cases, the symptoms can be so severe that even climbing stairs is impossible. The course is variable but the usual patient gets better with maturation of the skeleton.

The second pattern is directly related to trauma. A direct blow on the knee is usually the initiating event. Symptoms consist of retropatellar pain with activity. They may progress for several weeks after the initiating accident. The third group of patients have problems directly related to mechanical derangement of the patella. There is a sudden feeling of popping or slipping of the patella that occurs during an activity producing lateral rotation of the tibia or the femur. The knee usually buckles. There is usually an accompanying effusion, which resolves over a week or two.

In true lateral dislocation of the patella, a mass occurs on the lateral aspect of the knee with the knee held midway between flexion and extension. Reduction is accompanied by dramatic relief of pain followed by the rapid onset of an effusion, pain, and tenderness over the medial retinacular area. Complications such as an osteochondral fracture may occur. A surprising number of these patients find that their symptoms resolve completely after the initial episode and that they are then able to return to a relatively normal life unless recurrence of the dislocation supervenes.

Usually after the initial episode, the course tends to be progressive, marked with episodes of "giving way." The knee buckles, and the patient may fall. Knee pain then becomes more intense, lasting for a variable period of time before returning to the baseline level. "Locking" results from the knee being held in partial flexion by flexor muscle spasm. Pain during the last 30° of extension is characteristic. In many patients, even stair climbing becomes intolerable. Notably absent in the history are marked or tense effusion and pain at rest.

The examination usually shows a healthy individual. The gait may be normal or with a stiff knee in full extension, or mildly antalgic. Inspection with the patient standing may show lateral placement with the kneecap (frog's eyes) and flattening on the medial aspect of the patella where normally the vastus medialis bulge would be. The lateral position of the patella is accentuated in the sitting position.

Attempted extension of the knee against resistance reveals that there is a patellofemoral pain beginning at about 30° of flexion and continuing to nearly full extension. This finding is pathognomonic. If the patellar tendon is observed while the knee is extended against resistance, lateral angulation of the patellar tubercule can be seen. With the quadriceps relaxed, the knee is carefully evaluated for the presence of an effusion. In the chondromalacia patellae syndrome, the presence of significant effusion is uncommon. A tense effusion is almost never present. The patella is now gently manipulated over the femoral condyle.

Frequently painful, coarse crepitus can be elicited. Remember that asymptomatic patellofemoral crepitance may be found in 60% of the population under 25 years of age. If the patella is gently brought medially, with pressure by the thumb over its lateral aspect, the medial facet of the patella can be palpated. A tender area on the medical articular surface of the patella is a pathognomonic finding. If the patella is then forced laterally, the patient suddenly resists the maneuver and pushes the examiner's hand away. The patient usually states that he or she feels as if the patella is about to go "out of place" (patella apprehension sign). Tenderness along the joint line is uncommon and the knee is stable.

X-ray changes are uncommon. The films should be evaluated for increased subchondral bone density, patellar dysplasia, narrowing of the joint space, and fracture or osteophytes on the lateral margin of the patellae. Arthroscopy of the knee may reveal a normal joint surface despite significant pathology in the deeper cartilaginous layers.

Treatment is generally conservative until pain becomes severe. Patient education should emphasize avoiding stressful flexion activity of the knee such as climbing stairs, crouching, and prolonged sitting or standing. As restricted activities continue, isometric quadriceps exercises, but not resistance exercises, should be initiated to prevent atrophy and instability.

The mainstays of conservative therapy are aspirin, rest, and exercise. Corticosteroids, on the other hand, although they frequently produce dramatic relief of pain should be avoided.

In conjunction with salicylate therapy, the patient is begun on an exercise program for quadriceps strengthening. Isometric exercises and isokinetic exercises are carried out through the last 30° of knee extension. Flexion of the knee beyond 30° increases the compression of the patella against the femoral condyle and should be avoided.

In patients in whom symptomatic relief is not achieved by an exercise program and salicylates, or who present with severe patellofemoral pain initially, patellar stabilization with a brace (Figure 3–2), progressing to immobilization with a plaster cylinder if the patella immobilization brace is ineffective. During immobilization, isometric quadriceps exercises are essential to prevent atrophy of the vastus medialis and to allow cartilage nutrition by maintaining some degree of repetitive motion at the patellofemoral joint. The cylinder is allowed to remain in place for about 2 weeks, at which time it is removed and the patient is fitted with a flexible patellar support. The patient is then returned to the exercise program already described until skeletal maturity. The patellar brace is worn continuously at first and later only during athletics until complete skeletal maturity has been achieved.

With severe refractory symptoms, surgical intervention is often required and varies from conservative arthrotomy with shaving of the involved cartilage or femoral ridge to a patellectomy. As with many common disorders, the natural history is poorly documented, but is usually one of resolution after 2 years. Patients have only occasional flare-ups of symptoms. There is a suspicion, but no evidence, that patellofemoral osteoarthritis follows chondromalacia.

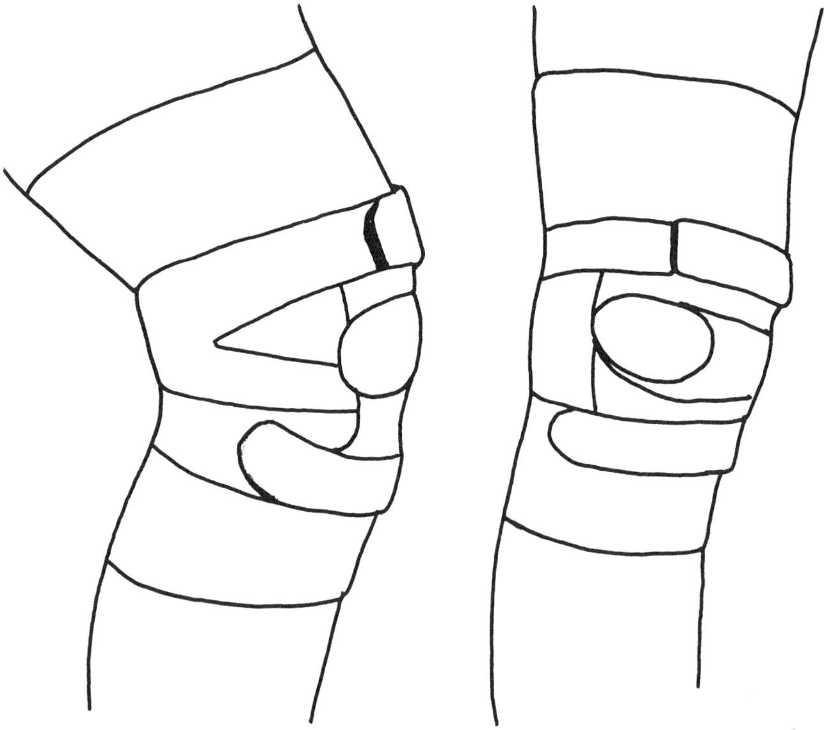

Figure 3–2. Patellar immobilizing brace.

REFERRED PAIN

When knee pain occurs without any physical findings, think of referred pain from the hip or an osseous lesion. Any painful condition of or near the hip may present as knee pain. Trochanteric bursitis, osteoarthritis of the hip, slipped femoral capital epiphysis, and infection are possibilities and are suggested by an abnormal examination of the hip. Osseous lesions either of the patella or the long bones contiguous with the knee can cause knee pain.

KNEE PAIN WITH EFFUSION

A joint effusion implies synovitis and points to a structure inside or next to the joint capsule as the cause of the problem. In the primary care setting, a small- to moderate-size effusion in the knees only is likely to be due to microtrauma to the meniscus or ligaments, viral illness, or, less frequently, to early rheumatoid arthritis or to the spondyloarthropathies.

One tends to think of ligament and meniscal problems as sports injuries, but minor trauma in the susceptible, older person can produce the same injury. The common precipitating factor is a twisting force to the knee with the foot planted. In the older person, an innocuous event such as stepping from a curb on a bus the wrong way can produce a meniscal tear.

With acute trauma, both ligamentous and meniscal injury may occur. In ligamentous injury, the swelling and tenderness is diffuse and imprecisely localized as compared to meniscus tears. In a severe meniscus tear, the knee may not extend and tests for joint stability are difficult to evaluate. In such cases or if there is suspicion of significant injury, a referral is the most appropriate course.

An accumulation of a joint effusion within 2 hours of injury, until proven otherwise, is a hemarthrosis; whereas, that which appears 12 to 24 hours after injury indicates a synovial effusion. Blood in the joint fluid suggests a traumatic internal derangement or a fracture. Fat globules in the joint fluid point to a fracture.

In examining the acutely painful knee for joint stability, test the normal knee first to establish a baseline and to demonstrate that you will not be rough. Most importantly, explain each step and apply stress very, very slowly to the point of pain. In this way, maximal laxity can be demonstrated without inducing muscle spasm. If suspicion for a ligamentous tear is great, parenteral analgesics or regional or general anesthesia may be needed to allow definitive examination. If the initial test is positive, but subsequent tests are negative because of pain and reflexive muscle spasm, assume that a ligament tear exists. If there is a suspicion that a tear is being masked by muscle spasm, immobilization in a cylinder cast will often relax the muscles and allow demonstration of joint laxity.

In correlating physical findings with operative findings, the following generalizations can be made: a) Complete disruption of the medial compartment of the knee may occur without significant pain, effusion, or disability for walking. b) The valgus stress test with the knee at 30° of flexion is a reliable indicator of a complete tear of the medial compartment. c) A positive valgus stress test at full extension is the most reliable clinical indication of an acute rupture of the posterior cruciate ligament in association with medial compartment disruption. d) A strongly positive anterior drawer sign with the tibia in external rotation indicates that the medial capsular, posterior oblique, and anterior cruciate ligaments are ruptured.

Lateral instability of the knee (acute and chronic) is infrequent but is often more disabling than medial instability of a comparable degree. Unfortunately, the clues for lateral instability are subtle and are frequently missed. Symptoms after acute injuries are usually no more than mild-to-moderate pain over the lateral joint line. Walking is not difficult and there is no sensation of instability. Persons may occasionally notice difficulty or instability when running or stopping suddenly.

Periodic exacerbations occur with ligamentous strains. These ligamentous lesions are minute and, unless they are superficial, are usually difficult to locate precisely.

A lax knee following ligamentous injury is a common cause of chronic disability. Examination will usually reveal quadriceps atrophy, and considerable improvement may result from muscle strengthening alone.

If stability is not impaired, conservative treatment includes splint bandaging of the knee, application of cold during the acute phase and heat in the convalescent period, graduated quadriceps exercise, and guarded resumption of activity. A satisfactory splint may be made with several thicknesses of bulky dressing underneath a firmly applied elastic bandage.

Accurate diagnosis of the acutely injured knee is important because specific treatment is dependent on the severity of the injury. An acute ligament tear can be repaired with good results, whereas a chronic tear may not be repaired satisfactorily and can lead to prolonged disability and discomfort. Even when instability of the joint is demonstrated, considerable clinical judgment is required for determining the need for an operation.

Diagnosis of meniscal tears, their conservative treatment, indications for arthroscopy, and meniscus surgery are discussed in the next section.

KNEE PAIN WITH LOCKING

Locking and giving way are symptoms that suggest interference with normal flexion and extension of the knee. They are uncommon symptoms in younger persons and suggest subluxation of the patella or lateral discoid meniscus. In adults, a torn meniscus or ligament, or loose body are diagnostic possibilities, but remember that one half of meniscal tears do not have locking as a symptom.

A consistent history of locking warrants an x-ray examination to look for radioopaque foreign bodies and magnetic resonance imaging (MRI), an arthrogram, or arthroscopy for definitive diagnosis. Magnetic resonance imaging is more effective in detecting small intrameniscal tears than an arthrogram but is twice as expensive. Due to its noninvasive nature, magnetic resonance imaging may become the procedure of choice for evaluation of possible meniscal lesions. Probing the surface of the cartilage allows an arthroscopist to detect significant intrameniscal tears that do not communicate with the surface. Consequently, when the history and physical strongly support the diagnosis of a meniscal tear, an arthroscopy may be needed eventually.

Meniscus injuries result from weight bearing upon the knee combined with faulty, forceful, or excessive motion, either in flexion rotation or extension rotation.

In the fully extended knee, no significant lateral or rotary motion is possible unless an overwhelming force tears the ligament or causes a fracture or dislocation. During a normal movement, flexion is accompanied by internal rotation of the tibia upon the femur and extension is accompanied by external rotation. The ligaments slacken or become taut with flexion, and the menisci move forward in extension and backward in flexion. Anatomically, the medial meniscus is firmly attached around its entire perimeter and moves less than the lateral meniscus, which is more centrally attached to the underlying bone. Therefore, by virtue of its greater mobility, the lateral meniscus sustains less injury. Factors such as ligamentous laxity, muscular inadequacy, and excessive knee valgus or varus may increase susceptibility to injury.

Meniscus injury is usually suggested by a history of trauma. The typical story is a blow against the lateral aspect of the knee with the knee flexed and the foot planted on the ground, or a twisting, turning movement of the leg with the foot planted or coming to an erect position from a full crouch. Seemingly trivial trauma in an older person may produce meniscal tears, and the history is less helpful in suspecting the proper diagnosis.

The pain is usually quite severe and sudden, and patients often describe that something tore within the knee. Pain intensity is such that activity is usually stopped, whereas pain from minor sprains permits continued activity although there is discomfort. After a meniscal tear, swelling occurs within hours.

Of the common tears of the semilunar cartilage, the bucket-handle tear is accompanied by locking and is relieved by surgery. Tears of the anterior or posterior horns, transverse tears of the middle portion, and horizontal fissures are compatible with continued function.

Locking is an important symptom, but nearly one-half of meniscal tears do not have such a history. Locking is rare when meniscal tears are restricted to the posterior third or if there is no displacement or bunching up of the cartilage. If a longitudinal tear is limited to the posterior third of the meniscus, the inherent elasticity of the meniscus allows it to spring back into a functional position. If the tear is extensive and goes past the collateral ligament anteriorly, the meniscus may bunch up between the two condyles and cause locking as a symptom. In extensive tears, the entire inner fragment may be forced to the center of the joint within the intercondylar fossa, in which case no locking results. True locking and unlocking is usually sudden. Gradual locking suggests a hemorrhagic effusion or a loose body within the joint.

Other symptoms of meniscal injury include buckling or giving way of the knee, which may be due to a tear of the posterior segment of the meniscus and/or quadriceps weakening. Clicking may also be noticed and is thought to be due to the femoral condyle riding over an irregularity of the articular surface. This sound also occurs in an osteoarthritic knee, in chondromalacia patellae, or when the hamstring tendon snaps over the femoral condyle.

A joint effusion is invariably present following the initial injury, although lesions of the lateral meniscus usually have a smaller effusion than lesions of the medial cartilage. Tenderness along the entire joint line points to tearing of the peripheral attachments of the meniscus. Tenderness is common in the posterior area of the knee joint. Pain along the joint line correlates well with operative findings of meniscus injury. In meniscus tear, tenderness may be in the region of the medial collateral ligaments, but tears of the ligament with or without meniscus injury cause tenderness above the joint line.

Compressing the articular surfaces by rotating the tibia on the femur will reproduce pain in meniscal injuries. Distracting the two bones while twisting the knee stresses the ligament and reproduces the pain of a ligamentous injury. These two physical examination tests can be done with the patient prone and the knee bent at 40°. The examiner applies force on the patient's foot bottom while rotating the tibia ("grind test") or, conversely, pulls up on the foot while stabilizing the femur to produce distraction at the knee. Since there are no nerve endings in the cartilage, pain results from stretching, tearing of the cartilaginous insertion of bone and periosteum, and acute synovial reaction within the joint space. Therefore, the severity of a meniscus injury does not parallel the severity of pain.

The McMurray test for meniscal tears is done with the knee flexed. The tibia is internally and externally rotated. Pain in either direction suggests a tear. Next, with the leg externally rotated and the knee with valgus stress, the knee is slowly entended. A palpable or audible click suggests a torn medial meniscus.

The definitive test is arthroscopy or arthrogram, which each necessitate a referral, or magnetic resonance imaging. Prices for these procedures are usually in a ratio 1:2:5, arthrogram: arthroscopy: MRF.

MENISCAL TEAR

Tears in the avascular portion of the fibrocartilage do not heal, whereas tears in the peripheral zone heal primarily by the invasion of fibrous tissue. Tears that do extend into the highly vascular peripheral area heal if there is a reduction of the displaced meniscus and the knee is immobilized for at least 3 weeks. In an obvious tear in which there is incomplete knee extension, indicating medial displacement of the meniscus, conservative treatment only delays the definitive treatment that is necessary to ensure pain-free return of function. Deciding when surgery is necessary is not easy and requires orthopedic surgical advice.

Meniscectomy should not be undertaken lightly. Cartilage regenerates but with a lesser quality biomaterial. Ten years after a meniscectomy, around 85% of patients will have degenerative changes of the knee. Pain, instability, locking, and painful catches on flexion are often reported. There is little evidence that leaving a torn meniscus will necessarily be harmful. More information about the natural history of meniscus injuries and the responses to conservative treatment is needed.

Conservative treatment is indicated if there is full extension of the knee and if locking is not present. A definitive diagnosis may not possible immediately following the injury. More careful examination may be possible after the effusion and acute pain have subsided.

PAIN IN THE HIP

Pain from the hip may be experienced as discomfort in the groin, buttock, or thigh. Each of these three patterns implies a separate differential diagnosis (Table 3–3). The more significant intraarticular causes of hip pain often present with anterior groin pain. The common causes of pain in the hip seen in the primary care setting are osteoarthritis and a variety of soft-tissue syndromes. In younger patients, pain in the thigh or knee associated with a limitation of the range of motion at the hip joint suggests Perthes' disease, slipped femoral capital epiphysis, inflammatory arthritis, congenital dislocation, or infection. In adults, hip pain is infrequently due to loose body in the hip joint, Paget's disease, infection, or aseptic necrosis.

TABLE 3–3. DIFFERENTIAL DIAGNOSIS OF HIP PAIN BY REGION*

Anterior Groin	Lateral	Buttock
Osteoarthritis (OA) — primary or secondary	Trochanteric bursitis	Muscular pain owing to strain or posture, tight hip flexors
Rider's (adductor) strain	Osteoarthritis	Osteoarthritis
Iliopsoas tendinitis	Tight fascia lata	Peripheral vascular disease
Iliopectineal bursitis	Radiating pain from back	Ischial bursitis
Hernia	Fracture	"Fibrositis nodules," tender points, trigger points
Ureteral stone	Meralgia paresthetica (lateral femoral cutaneous nerve entrapment)	Radiation from back
Fracture	Bone tumor	Sciatic nerve irritation from trauma or sitting
Septic joint		Sacroiliitis (spondyloarthropathy)
Inflammatory synovitis (rheumatoid arthritis, ankylosing spondylitis, systemic lupus, etc.)		
Aseptic necrosis of the femoral head		
Loose body		
Bone tumor		

TABLE 3–4. HIP (GROIN, BUTTOCK, THIGH) PAIN SYNDROMES

Abnormal Exam (Painful or Limited Range of Motion)
Infection of hip
Fracture
Osteoarthritis
Soft-tissue contractures
Tumor
Inflammatory arthritis
Bleeding
Charcot joint
Loose body
Retroperitoneal pathology
Normal Exam (Normal Range of Motion)
Bursitis/tendinitis
Early osteoarthritis
Bilateral involvement
Referred (lumbar spine, retroperitoneal space, knee)
Vascular insufficiency
Osseous lesion (Paget's aseptic necrosis, tumor, etc.)
Children
Congenital hip dislocation
Slipped femoral epiphyses
Tumor
Infection

Diagnostic Strategy

In children, hip, groin, or buttock pain is so unusual that they should always be x-rayed. Any child found limping or complaining of thigh or knee pain who shows a limitation of movement at the hip should be x-rayed. Possible diagnoses are Perthes' disease, slipped femoral capital epiphysis coxa vara, congenital dislocation of the hip, infection, or tumor — all requiring referral. The rest of this discussion is organized around two major clinical groups: hip (groin, buttock, or thigh) pain with an abnormal examination and hip pain with a normal examination (Table 3–4).

Most hip pain can be sorted out with a history and a limited physical examination. The history focuses on the pattern of onset, aggravating activities, and the quality of the pain (the latter to exclude ischemic or neurogenic pain). A limited examination of the hip and joints above (lumbar spine and sacroiliac joint) excludes referred pain and pinpoints areas of tenderness. If there is a symmetric, full, and painless range of rotation, the hip joint is almost certainly not the source of pain (Figure 3–3). When the range of motion is full and painless, think of early osteoarthritis, bilateral hip disease with symmetric findings or an "almost normal" examination, referred pain (usually from the back), arterial insufficiency, or an osseous lesion. If the hip has limited or a painful range of motion, or if a point of discrete tenderness can be identified, the diagnoses listed in Table 3–3 are possibilities.

On the initial visit, one should not miss a septic hip, a fracture, referred pain

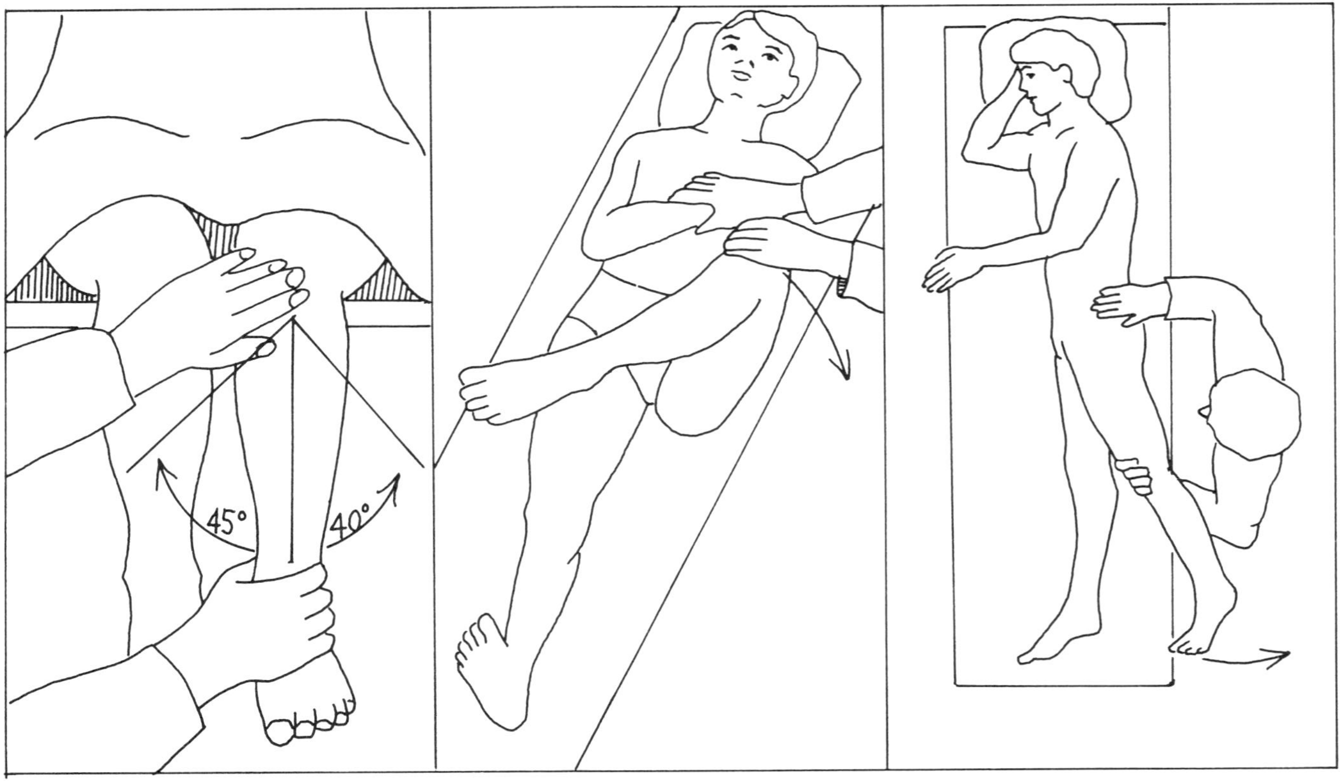

Figure 3–3. Examination of the hip. Symmetric, full, painless internal (ankle out) and external (ankle in) rotation of the hip in a sitting position effectively rules out intraarticular hip disease (Panel A). In contrast, common findings in osteoarthritis of the hip are groin pain on rotation or on the FABER (*f*lexion, *a*bduction, *e*xternal *r*otation) maneuver (Panel B) and, in early disease, asymmetrically restricted hip extension (Panel C).

TABLE 3–5. HIP (GROIN, BUTTOCK, OR THIGH) PAIN — DON'T MISS

Fracture
Infection
In children
Legg–Perthes
congenital hip dislocation
slipped femoral capital epiphyses
Herniated disc

from retroperitoneal pathology, or a herniated disc with nerve-root compression — all conditions that may present with hip, buttock, groin, or thigh pain (Table 3–5).

Pain History

The cardinal feature suggesting intraarticular hip disease is groin pain in the history or on the physical exam. The hip joint forms largely from the third lumbar segment, and thus pain is referred from the groin, from the front of the thigh to the knee, and down the front of the leg to just above the ankle. The upper inner quadrant of the buttock is also part of the third lumbar dermatome and hip pathology frequently hurts here. Occasionally, a patient will complain only of a unilateral backache when the hip is the problem. Another presentation of a hip problem is knee pain alone. When the examination of the hip and back is completely normal, the knee may be the source. Rarely, the hip joint develops within the fourth lumbar segment, and thus hip pain may spread to the outer side of the midthigh and leg, and may resemble sciatica. Pain felt only at the anterior thigh may arise from the lumbar spine, the hip joint, the thigh muscles themselves, or the knee. Specific historical clues sometimes hint at the diagnosis (Table 3–6).

Physical Examination (Fig 3–3)

The hip joint is examined by taking the hip through a full range of motion: flexion, abduction, and external rotation with the hip in flexion (the FABER maneuver). The extremes of passive flexion and internal/external rotation have a "hard end feel" in osteoarthritis, and this is quite different from the "soft end feel" of bursitis or synovitis. In these latter disorders early on, there is no gross limitation of flexion, abduction, or internal rotation, and only slight or no limitation of extension and lateral or external rotation.

Contractures of the hip are detected by the Thomas test. The patient is supine and the lordosis is eliminated by flexing the other hip. The extent of a flexion contracture is roughly the angle between the bed and the patient's leg. Leg-length discrepancy is also sought. Beware that the hip joint is deep, and joint effusions are impossible to detect by physical examination alone.

TABLE 3–6. RED FLAGS IN DIAGNOSIS OF HIP PAIN

History	Condition
Recent fall, old age, osteoporosis	Fracture
Prepubertal or adolescent	Dysplasia, infection, congenital dislocation
Abrupt onset, fever, immunosuppression, pain at rest	Septic joint
Subacute onset, oral corticosteroids, systemic lupus, alcoholism, hemodialysis	Avascular necrosis
History of other arthritis	Inflammatory synovitis (e.g., rheumatoid arthritis, spondyloarthropathy, etc.)
History of cancer	Bone metastasis

If trunk extension causes buttock ache, the pain cannot be from the muscles, as this motion relaxes the sacrospinalis and gluteal muscles. However, the movement stresses the lumbar, hip, and sacroiliac joint and the psoas muscle group. Thus, pain evoked by trunk extension is articular or retroperitoneal until proven otherwise. When buttock pain is produced by resisted extension of the hip, pathology in the gluteal muscles and psoas (retroperitoneal site) is suspected.

HIP PAIN WITH ABNORMAL EXAM

Osteoarthritis of the Hip

The symptoms of early osteoarthritis of the hip are pain and stiffness that is worse after activity or weight bearing. Pain or stiffness is most commonly referred to the region of the greater trochanter (in about 60% of the cases) and to the knee, back of the thigh, groin, and buttock in the remaining percentage.

Depending on the clinical criteria and the population surveyed, the prevalence of this condition varies from 3.5% to 20% of the adult population. Danielson, from an examination of the x-rays of 3903 patients with normal barium enema studies, found 3.5% to have osteoarthritis of the hip using strict diagnostic criteria. The prevalence was equal in males and females; one third of the patients had disease in both hips.

Danielson has made observations of the natural history of osteoarthritis of the hip relevant to our understanding of the disease. In his study, the presence or absence of osteophytes was excluded as a criterion for the diagnosis of osteoarthritis. These criteria are in marked contrast to those of most physicians, who would make the diagnosis based on the appearance of osteophytes alone. Danielson's definition is supported by observations on a subset of 86 patients in whom the diagnosis of osteoarthritis of the hip was made solely on the presence of osteophytes without joint-space narrowing. Over an 11-year follow-up, these persons had a benign course, only one showing joint-space narrowing and the rest having no deterioration of the joint. Likewise, Lloyd–Roberts could find no clear relationship between osteophytes and the symptoms experienced by patients.

The earliest definable x-ray lesion of hip osteoarthritis is unequal narrowing of the joint space. On a routine view of the pelvis, the width should be the same in both hips, and minor narrowing may be picked up if the normal side is compared to the affected side. If bilateral narrowing is present, a greater degree or narrowing must be present before the diagnosis can be made with confidence. The joint space is probably abnormal if it is less than 4 mm in patients under age 70 or less than 3 mm in patients over 70. When compared to the contralateral side, the joint space is "abnormal" if it is more than 1 mm different in width.

Osteoarthritis of the hip is divided into primary and secondary types. Idiopathic or primary osteoarthritis of the hip can be classified into two or more distinct groups according to the pattern of damage seen on the radiograph. The two major types of osteoarthritis, superolateral and medial, account for the majority of cases (Table 3–7). Clinically, these subsets are useful for predicting the course of the disorder. With superolateral disease, persistent unilateral involvement is the rule. On examination, decreased internal rotation of the hip with or without pain is the earliest sign of disease. In advanced disease, loss of motion may become manifest in other directions and the hip is abducted, flexed, and foreshortened.

In the unusual "medial" form of osteoarthritis, the joint space lost is more equally narrowed. Sinking of the acetabular floor may produce a picture of protursio acetabuli. In this form, lateral and rotational movements are decreased more or less equally and, although flexion deformity often develops, the hip remains in an approximately neutral position and a useful range of flexion is usually maintained. In osteoarthritis with predominant medial joint-space narrowing, involvement is usually bilateral when initially seen or becomes bilateral with follow-up.

Secondary osteoarthritis of the hip implies antecedent conditions that are predisposing or sufficient causes for the degenerative process. Secondary osteoarthritis may follow fractures of the upper femur or acetabulum or may be late sequela of childhood dysplasias such as slipped femoral capital epiphysis or Perthes' disease. Other minor dysplasias may also predispose to degenerative change. A condition known as congenital subluxation of the hip is thought to be a developmental abnormality of the hip involving the acetabulum, the head of the femur, or its neck. The anatomy resembles, to a minor degree, changes found in congenital dislocation of the hip. Estimates of the prevalence of this condition in osteoarthritic hips vary between 13% and 48% and reflect the difficulty in establishing this disease in advanced cases of osteoarthritis as well as case selection. Whether femoral head subluxation in osteoarthritic hips is primary or secondary to the remodeling process that occurs as disease progresses is unknown. Some believe that this dysplasia leads to osteoarthritis by age 50 to 60, but patients have been reported who have no osteoarthritic changes with this dysplasia.

For the generalist, identification of such patients may aid in understanding the natural history of the disease but is unlikely to indicate any specific manage-

TABLE 3–7. TYPES OF OSTEOARTHRITIS OF THE HIP

Types	Radiological Criteria	Characteristics
Superolateral	Narrowing of the joint space occurs first in the superolateral segment	Medial, lateral, and inferior osteophytes common. Femoral head tends to flatten as disease progresses. Sclerosis, pseudocysts, and femoral head collapse seen in advanced disease. Usually unilateral
Medial	Joint space narrowing occurs medially	The femoral head usually becomes deeply seated and protrusio-acetabuli of varying degrees may develop. Medial osteophyte not seen, but small peripheral osteophytes may be present. Usually bilateral.
Superomedial	Joint space narrowing begins medial to the lateral margin	Peripheral osteophytes, a buttress and femoral head distortion may occur. Unilateral or bilateral

ment. Since the natural history of congenital subluxation is unknown, surgical intervention is unwarranted.

Osteoarthritis of the Hip and Length Discrepancy

A potential cause of secondary osteoarthritis is leg-length discrepancy. In a study of leg-length inequality in patients with idiopathic osteoarthritis, over half were found to have had joint space narrowing first in the superiolateral segment of the joint. Measurements of the functional leg length of these 36 patients showed significant leg-length discrepancy, and most of the diseased hips were found on the side of the longer leg. Even when allowance was made for shortening due to disease, the frequency and bias of the disparity in leg lengths was highly significant.

Since the leg on the involved side is generally shortened by disease, the finding of a longer leg on the diseased side suggests that perhaps greater disparity existed before the onset of disease. A significant difference in leg length of more than one inch could impose stresses on the hip, which contribute to degenerative changes in the joint.

Leg length is commonly measured by taking the distance between the anterior superior iliac spine to the medial malleolus, but minor changes in the angle of the pelvis can change the measurement considerably. Probably more accurate is the functional leg length of the standing patient.

To take this measurement, the patient stands with the knees straight, the pelvis centered, and the feet parallel and about seven inches apart. The examiner sits behind the subject and is able to make three observations if there are differences between the leg lengths:

1. The upper lateral thigh on the long side will protrude.
2. Scoliosis will be apparent.
3. The examiner's hands placed on top of the iliac crest will rest at different heights.

This method can easily detect a difference of one-half inch between the two legs.

To confirm this impression, a block of appropriate thickness (¼ to ½ inch) should be placed under the foot of the presumed short side. At this point, the thighs should be symmetrical, the spine straight, and the hands level. Final confirmation is done by placing the same block under the presumed longer leg. The three original observations should now be exaggerated. The size of the block necessary to bring the pelvis to an appropriate level is an indication of the amount of disparity.

Obese and muscular patients will confound this technique as the hands cannot be placed on top of the iliac crest, nor can scoliosis be detected easily. Furthermore, a subject who cannot take the posture described above, or who has fixed deformities of the hip or knee, cannot be measured by this technique.

The basic principles in the management of the osteoarthritic hip have been described under Osteoarthritis of the Knee. Periodic exacerbations must be similarly distinguished from treatable causes of hip, groin, and buttock pain: bursitis (trochanteric, ischial), vascular insufficiency, tendinitis, synovitis, infection, and leg-length discrepancy.

Bursitis, Tendinitis, and Other Soft-Tissue Lesions

A variety of soft-tissue lesions (bursitis and tendinitis) about the hip may cause "hip pain." These can be the result of a primary joint problem or may occur as an isolated disorder or as the result of altered biomechanics or posture from joint disease elsewhere.

Osteoarthritis of the hip may present as pain in the area of the greater trochanter in about two-thirds of the cases. In many instances, trochanteric bursitis may be present. Palpation of the buttock superior to the greater trochanter reveals localized tenderness over the trochanteric bursa or at the insertion of the abductor tendons. If persistent adduction towards a long leg imposes greater stress on the hip, then increased force should also be exerted by the abductor muscles when the weight is borne on that leg. Thus, in leg-length discrepancy with or without degenerative changes in the hip, trochanteric bursitis and abductor muscle insertion tenderness are also frequent findings.

Rider's sprain or a sprain of the adductor muscles is diagnosed by asking the patient to squeeze the examiner's fist between the patient's knees. If this resisted adduction causes pain at the inner upper thigh, the upper extent of the adductor muscles has been strained at their insertion. Localized tenderness identifies the site of the lesion. Pain on resisted adduction is also elicited in fracture or neoplastic invasion of the os pubis. Therefore, if no tenderness of the muscles can be found on resisted adduction, an x-ray should be taken of the pubic bone. Occasionally, resisted adduction of the thigh hurts in the buttock, and this may point to lesions in the sacroiliac joint. Slight discomfort in resistive flexion may be felt in tendinitis of the rectus femoris or in tears of the upper extent of the quadriceps muscle. To test for these, resisted extension of the knee should be done while the patient is lying prone in order to maintain extension at the hip. Soft-tissue lesions respond to massage, heat, and/or injections of local anesthetics and corticosteroid agents (Figure 3–4). In patients with leg-length discrepancy of greater than an inch, a heel lift to the shorter leg would normalize the distribution of weight on the hip joints and might possibly prevent progression of disease in the long leg. Immediate or long-term benefit is unproven, but a trial with a lift can do no harm.

HIP PAIN WITH NORMAL EXAMINATION

Hip (groin, buttock, or thigh) pain associated with a normal examination of the hip joint and no areas of discrete tenderness suggests that the pain is referred or is from bilateral hip disease (Table 3–4). Early osteoarthritis or inflammatory arthritis has few or no physical findings. Bilateral involvement eliminates the use of the "normal side" as a control and thus gives the appearance of a normal examination. Referred pain from the joints above and below the hip joint has

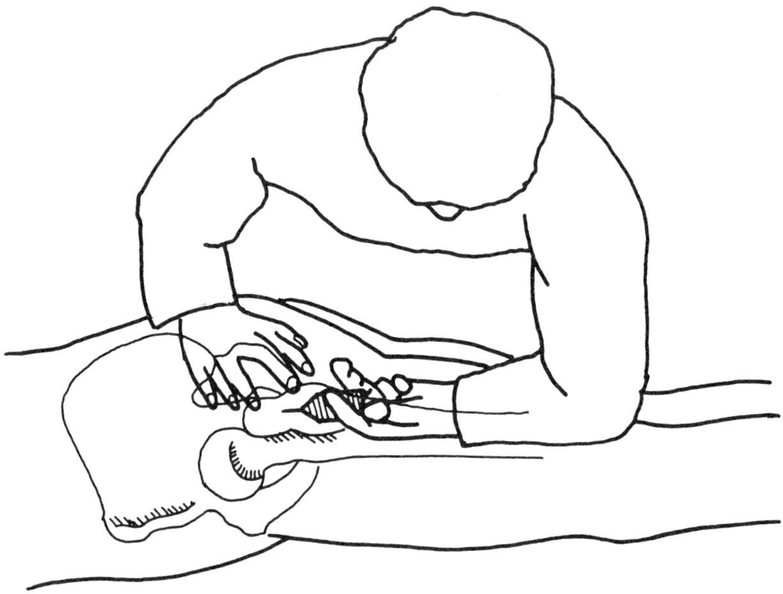

Figure 3–4. Trochanteric bursa injection. The needle enters at 90° to the skin and is aimed at the point of maximal tenderness. The needle should be advanced to bone then withdrawn slightly before injection.

fooled the most experienced physician. In patients who complain of hip pain and have no apparent physical findings, one should always check the knee and the lumbar spine. Finally, when the anatomical site of the pain is unknown, the pain bears no relationship to weight bearing, or the person is under 20 or over 45 years, an x-ray of the area will have a high diagnostic yield for an osseous lesion.

Tumor

In general medical practice, malignant tumors or new growths that develop as primary lesions in the skeletal system are exceedingly rare. Less rare are benign non-neoplastic lesions and metastatic bone lesions. For the generalist, it is more important to learn about the general features and their clinical presentation rather than differential diagnosis or specific treatment of bone tumors.

Many tumors develop during childhood at the sites of greatest bone turnover, in the metaphyseal regions of the lower femur, and in the tibia and upper humerus, areas that might present as knee or shoulder pain. Thus, joint pain in children, especially when there are no objective signs of synovitis or obvious explanations, is cause for worry. Slow-growing bone tumors and benign lesions of the bone seldom cause pain unless it stretches the endosteum or periosteum or has fractured. Pain from neoplasms becomes more constant and unrelated to use.

Once the diagnosis of an osseous lesion is suspected, an x-ray of the region and/or NMRI or a bone scan is needed. The radiographic appearance reliably differentiates benign from malignant lesions and distinguishes primary versus secondary (metastatic) disease. Neoplasms do not destroy bone but stimulate local osteoclastic resorption of reactive bone and new bone formation. In slow-growing lesions, periosteal new bone formation gives the appearance of expansion of the bone. When the periosteum is elevated by neoplasm that has eroded the cortex, it produces reactive bone in the angle where the periosteum is still attached, *Codman's triangle*. If the lesion is a primary bone tumor, without clinical evidence of spread from another primary, it must have a tissue diagnosis and clinical staging of its extent, both of which are most efficiently done in the hospital with consultation. If the lesion is metastatic, then it is by definition an advanced tumor, usually thyroid, breast, kidney, or prostate. The workup is best done in the hospital setting.

HIP PAIN IN CHILDREN

Perthes' Disease (Legg-Calve-Perthes' Disease)

Perthes' disease is an idiopathic avascular necrosis of the femoral epiphysis. As with other osteochondroses, it is most common during the middle years of growth from the ages of three to ten, is more common in boys than girls, and is bilateral in about 15% of those affected. Approximately 5% of children with transient synovitis of the hip develop the complication of Perthes' disease.

The disease is usually quiet during the early phase of necrosis, and it is not until later that pain is felt in the region of the hip or is occasionally referred to the knee. At this point, the lesion is advanced. On examination, there is limited abduction and internal rotation. Disuse atrophy is most prominent in the upper thigh muscles. The child walks with a limp to protect against pain by rapidly taking weight off the foot on the involved side with each step. The diagnosis can only be suspected clinically, and a bone scan or NMRI is needed for diagnosis of the earliest lesion.

Osteochondrosis is a self-limited disease unless secondary osteoarthritis occurs. The principal aim of management is to prevent deformity of the epiphysis, thus preserving joint function and preventing secondary osteoarthritis. Perthes' disease may be complicated by subchondral fracture of the epiphysis, subluxation of the joint, flattening of the epiphysis with resulting incongruity, and late degenerative joint disease. Treatment requires specialized experience and is directed towards preventing abnormal forces on the femoral head during its vulnerable phase of revascularization and bony healing. It is likely that children aged three to four with only partial resorption of the femoral head will have a good result without treatment. In contrast, most children with resorption of the entire head and those over the age of four who have resorption of only a part of the head should be treated by non-weight bearing and an abduction plaster cast or some type of abduction brace, both of which prevent subluxation and enable the acetabulum to mold the healing femoral head in such a way that it does not become deformed. Surgical operations are also available for the older child who has previously had a bad prognosis, provided the operation is done before any deformity has developed.

More than in any other osteochondroses, the prognosis of Perthes' disease, even with treatment, is extremely variable. The age of onset or detection is an important factor and, in general, the earlier the diagnosis, the better the prognosis.

Slipped Femoral Epiphysis (adolescent coxa vara)

The upper femoral epiphysis lies oblique to the axis of the femoral shaft and is extremely vulnerable to shearing force. Any weakness of the epiphyseal plate, even with normal weight bearing, may cause the femoral head to slip off the neck. Such slippage is most likely to occur in children beginning at age nine to the end of active growth and in tall, thin, rapidly growing adolescents. Although usually unilateral, there is a one in three chance that the opposite site will become involved as well. The etiology of the condition is not known.

The epiphysis usually slips insidiously and leads to progressive coxa vera deformity with secondary remodeling of the femoral neck. Acute injury superimposed on this process may cause further slippage or complete separation, thus compromising the already precarious blood supply of the femoral head, leading to avascular necrosis. Once the epiphysis closes at puberty, no further slip occurs, but residual displacement of the femoral head alters the mechanics of the hip and leads to degenerative disease of the hip in adult life.

Early diagnosis is of extreme importance so that treatment may be instituted in the earliest stages of slipping. The most common presenting complaint, mild discomfort in the hip or referred pain to the knee, is deceptively innocent. A slight limp may occasionally be noticed. With progressive slippage, the affected limb becomes externally rotated. On examination, the hip is limited on internal rotation and abduction. The diagnosis is made positively by radiographic examination of the femur in an anteroposterior view and lateral projection, the latter demonstrating a minimal slip more clearly.

Treatment

The treatment of slipped epiphysis is surgery and requires referral to an orthopedist skilled in the problems of children.

Slipping of the epiphysis constantly threatens the blood supply of the femoral head. The aim of management is early detection and surgical stabilization of slips less than 1 cm in the lateral projection. This is accomplished by pinning the head. A chronic slip that has gone beyond 1 cm is much more difficult and requires surgical correction of the deformity, a procedure that carries the risk of causing iatrogenic avascular necrosis.

The follow-up care of children treated for slipped epiphysis continues until the epiphyseal plate closes. During this time, the opposite hip must be watched carefully because it has a one in three chance of slipping.

Congenital Dislocation of the Hip (CHD)

Congenital dislocation of the hip, an abnormality of the hip in which the femoral head lies outside the acetabulum but is still inside the capsule, occurs once every 1000 live births. The abnormality is bilateral in over half the children affected and is eight times more prevalent in girls than boys. In newborns, congenital dislocation of the hip may be detected by simple physical examination. Left undiagnosed and untreated, it leads inevitably to degenerative arthritis of the hip. It is uncommon for the generalist to see children over 5 years of age with previously untreated hip dislocation. This is fortunate since secondary degenerative changes in a complete dislocation are so marked and irreversible by this age that only salvage procedures or total joint replacements are possible. An occasional child will be diagnosed with partial subluxation of the hip in which the femoral head rides on the edge of the acetabulum. Subluxation or dislocation must be considered if a child complains of hip, groin, buttock, or knee pain, or limps. The examination shows the signs of abduction contracture: a limp, limitation of passive abduction, shortening of the involved leg, and prominence of the hip. The longer a hip has remained out of joint, the more difficult it is to feel the hip dislocate with the fixed hip abducted slightly while lifting the femur upward (the Ortolani test). Similarly, a subluxation cannot be felt at all.

When the child stands on one foot on the side of the dislocated hip, the hip abducters, having no fulcrum, cannot hold the pelvis level and the pelvis drops on the opposite side (a positive Trendelenburg sign). When the dislocation is unilateral, the child's gait looks as if he or she has a short leg on the side of the dislocation and shifts the trunk toward the involved side when weight is borne on that side. With bilateral dislocation, the child shifts the trunk from one side to the other, giving the impression of waddling. In subluxation, the Trendelenburg sign and gait disturbances are only apparent when the muscles are fatigued.

The treatment of dislocation or subluxation requires considerable experience and referral to an orthopedic surgeon specializing in problems of children.

PAINFUL FEET

Painful conditions of the foot commonly originate in the soft-tissue structures (the skin, muscles, ligaments, tendons, and bursae). Congenital deformity of the osseous structures or arthritis, trauma, or infection of the joints may cause pain, but even in these conditions, a large component of the pain comes from the soft tissue.

Common foot conditions are diagnosed by history and examination. The painful area identified by the patient usually specifies the anatomical site. Referred pain, such as heel pain referred from entrapment of the posterior tibial nerve and its calcaneal branch or from irritation of the S1 nerve root from a lumbar disc, is unusual. X-rays of the feet are of little diagnostic or therapeutic value in the initial management of most complaints. The joints are poorly visualized and alignment is difficult to interpret. The foot suffers considerable trauma, and osteophytes are common and are frequently unrelated to symptoms. The radiograph can confirm the diagnosis of fracture, aseptic necrosis, osteomyelitis, developmental anomalies, and some forms of inflammatory arthropathy, but other clinical information will suggest the possible diagnosis first. If foot pain persists or no specific diagnosis can be made, an x-ray can be helpful.

The type of pain is helpful. Acute or subacute pain suggests fracture, tendon rupture, crystal synovitis, or infection. Pain after prolonged use implies muscle, ligament, or tendon strain. Numbness and burning are qualities of neurogenic pain. Pain at rest occurs as a result of ischemia, neuropathy, or bursitis.

All the significant elements of the foot are accessible by inspection or feel. The patient's shoes give diagnostic and therapeutic clues. A normal foot and gait wears down the heel on the lateral edge and is an indication that the calcaneous is in the neutral position, the heel is centrally placed, and the foot is slightly inverted. The everted foot distorts the counter and wears the heel on its inner border. A shorter Achilles tendon tends to wear out the toe of the shoe. The worn areas of the sole indicate the position of the metatarsal heads.

The range of motion is tested during the examination of the bare foot. When the knee is straight, the gastrocnemius muscle, which originates above the knee and crosses the ankle joint, is stretched. Flexing the knee eliminates this and allows for a full range of motion. The range of motion should be judged from excursion of the hind foot, rather than the forefoot, so that movement of the longitudinal arch is not mistaken for ankle movement.

The subtalar joint is tested by holding the lower leg firmly and holding the heel with the ankle dorsiflexed, which fixes the ankle mortice and prevents lateral motion. Moving the heel from side to side represents movement at the talocalcaneal (subtalar) joint. Involvement of the joint may also be inferred by tenderness over the sinus tarsus in front of the lateral malleolus. Plantar tingling or numbness brought on or made worse by pressure over the neurovascular bundle containing the tibial nerve is diagnostic of tarsal tunnel syndrome. The bundle is most conveniently compressed just dorsal to the medial malleolus or over the sinus tarsus.

Metatarsal movement is tested by grasping the heel firmly with one hand and the forefoot at the base of the metatarsals with the other hand. Passive pronation and supination, and adduction and abduction of the forefoot assesses the range of motion.

The range of motion of the metatarsophalangeal joint of the big toe is 90° dorsiflexion, and 60° or less is abnormal. The big toe bears the brunt of normal walking and is the site of many painful conditions such as hallus valgus, hallux rigidus, bunion, osteoarthritis, or gout.

TABLE 3–8. FOOT PAIN

Painful Foot with Abnormal Exam

Plantar Surface	Toes	Heel	Ankle
Wart	Osteoarthritis	Plantar fasciitis	Strain
Callous	Hallux valgus	Painful heel pad	Sprain
Strain	Hallus rigidus	Achilles tendon rupture	Fracture
	Gout	Subtalar arthritis	Periositis
	Metatarsalgia	Fracture	Infection
	Arterial insufficiency		
	Infection		
	Fracture		

Painful Foot, No Findings of Joints or Soft Tissue

Plantar Surface	Toe(s)
Posterior tibial nerve entrapment (tarsal tunnel syndrome)	Arterial insufficiency
Referred	Interdigital nerve entrapment
	Anterior tibial nerve

TABLE 3–9. FOOT PAIN — DON'T MISS

Infection
Acute anterior compartment syndrome
(Acute arterial insufficiency)
Fracture
Internal derangement
(Torn ligament)
Crystal synovitis

Palpation of the pedal arteries should never be omitted. One or both dorsal pedal pulses may be absent in up to 12% of normal patients. Neurological testing begins with motor testing. The dorsiflexors (L4, L5, S1) of the foot and ankle may be tested simply by having the patient walk on the heels: difficulty (lurching) or inability indicates involvement of the deep peroneal branch, ligamentous abnormalities, gastroc-soleus contractures, or ankle joint disease (the latter being excluded by a normal passive range of motion of the ankle). The gastroc-soleus and the plantar flexors (L5, S1, S2) of the foot are so powerful that the only true test of strength is to have the patient rise on the tip toes of each foot repetitively. The knee and ankle deep tendon reflexes and a quick check of the sensory dermatomes and the Babinski sign complete the exam.

In summary, with attention to the nature of the pain, its mode of onset, modifying factors, and a directed examination, foot pain complaints can be quickly sorted into three major diagnostic groupings by considering which region of the foot is involved (Table 3–8). Do not miss diagnosing the treatable disorders listed in Table 3–9.

CHRONIC FOOT PAIN WITH ABNORMAL EXAMINATION

Corns, Calluses, and Plantar Warts

Corns are hyperkeratotic lesions of the plantar surface between the fourth and fifth toe that arise from constant pressure. If kept moist, the lesion cannot become cornified into a callus. A soft corn need not be treated unless it points to altered foot dynamics. When it is painful, it should be treated like a callus.

A callus is thickened skin in an area exposed to abnormal pressure or friction. Normal callus forms lie at the points of a triangle between the heel, the first toe, and the fifth toe. Altered foot mechanics produce calluses in other regions. When weight is borne primarily by the metatarsal heads, plantar calluses develop. In the inverted foot, a callus appears under the fifth metatarsal head. If the toes are clawed, their knuckles develop calluses where pressed against the shoe.

Calluses are differentiated from their look-alikes (plantar warts) by four characteristics. Calluses and corns have normal skin prints running over their surface; warts do not. If one squeezes a corn with lateral pressure, it does not hurt but a wart does. Calluses have a well-demarcated, translucent, avascular core; warts have darker centers with capillaries running perpendicular to the surface. The core of a wart can be stretched from the surrounding skin leaving a cleft. A variant of corns, the neurovascular corn, occurs over bony prominences and is sharply demarcated. It has small blood vessels that lie parallel to the surface.

Corns and calluses are usually benign except for the altered foot dynamics that they suggest. The important exceptions are diabetics, persons with arterial insufficiency, or sensory deficits. In such individuals, do not miss providing foot care to prevent infection and skin breakdown. A corn or callus with a deep hemorrhagic area is troublesome and should be followed very closely: Skin breakdown is inevitable.

Corns and calluses are treated with topical 40% salicylic acid, plaster, and a doughnut pad to prevent further pressure or friction. Definitive treatment consists of preventing abnormal contact with the shoe or correcting abnormal foot mechanics with orthotics or altered shoes.

Plantar warts are very troublesome to treat. There have been no controlled trials. Warts have been attacked with curettage, cautery, radiotherapy, liquid nitrogen, and surgery. The object is not to cause more harm (scarring or infection) than good. Conservative treatment consists of repeated applications of salicylic acid and time.

TOE PAIN

Pain in the Great Toe

The common causes of chronic or indolent pain in the first metatarsophalangeal (MTP) joint is osteoarthritis, hallus valgus, hallus rigidus, and gout (podagra).

Acute, subacute, and severe toe pain is almost certainly crystalline synovitis (usually gout) or infection. Pseudogout (synovitis induced by deposition of calcium pryphosphate crystals) is rare in the first metatarsophalangeal joint.

Hallux Valgus

Hallux valgus is the most common painful condition of the big toe. At the stage when the patient seeks relief, three components are present: a) the large toe drifts laterally, b) the medial portion of the first metatarsal enlarges, and c) the bursa over the medial aspect of the metatarsophalangeal joint is inflamed.

Many patients with severe deformity have no symptoms; others with minimal changes need treatment. In the elderly patient, conservative treatment is often satisfactory. Molded shoes, sandals, etc. prevent pressure on the protruded portions of the foot. In the middle-aged person, attention to restoring the longitudinal and transverse arches, bunion pads, and roomy shoes are helpful and should always proceed surgery. By one count, there are 78 different procedures for the correction of this deformity; many are variations on the theme and only about 20 are commonly used. In any case, pain relief is achieved in about 85% of the patients who undergo surgery but no controlled experience has been reported.

Hallus Rigidus

Hallus rigidus or less severe hallux limitus or inflexibility of the metatarsophalangeal joint of the big toe is the second most common cause of a painful toe. Since every step requires pushing off with the big toe, restriction of joint motion causes pain. With time, persistent inflammation leads to ankylosis and pain may disappear. The patient with hallus rigidus frequently complains of pain elsewhere in the foot resulting from attempts to avoid pain in the toe. Conservative but unproven treatment consists of a shoe with a wide forefoot, which permits the forefoot to adduct, and a metatarsal pad under and behind the first metatarsal head. Another alternative is a steel shank in the sole of the shoe beneath the affected metatarsophalangeal joint to prevent the shoe from bending at that point so that no force is transmitted directly to the metatarsophalangeal joint. Surgery, when symptoms are severe, usually consist of resection of the joint and remodeling of the metatarsal head.

Crystal-Induced Synovitis

Crystal synovitis, usually gout and rarely pseudogout, comes on and looks like an infection, the major differential diagnosis. The pain is acute and severe. The toe is red, swollen, warm, and painful to touch and to the slightest motion.

Both forms of crystal synovitis present as subacute or acute arthritis attacks whose natural history is approximately days to 4 weeks. The episodes are self-limited and generally involve one joint or a few joints. The average pseudogout attack takes longer to reach peak intensity and is somewhat less painful and disabling. Inflammation may begin in one joint, and acute attacks postoperative-

TABLE 3–10. CAUSES OF METATARSALGIA

Flattening of the transverse arch
Stress (pes cavus, pronated feet)
March fracture of the metatarsal shaft
Plantar keratosis
Frieberg's disease (osteochondritis of metatarsal)

ly or during medical illness (with fluid shifts or dehydration) are common to both gout and pseudogout. Positive diagnosis of crystal synovitis is made by joint aspiration. The fluid is characteristically inflammatory with poor stringing and shows sheets of polymorphonuclear leucocytes with ingested crystals.

Urate may be distinguished from calcium pyrophosphate by compensated polarized microscopy. Urate crystals are needle-shaped and show strongly negative birefringence on polarizing microscopy. With a first-order red compensator, urate appears yellow when the axis of the crystal is parallel to the compensator. Calcium pyrophosphate crystals are much more pleomorphic than urate and appear as a weakly positive birefringence, nonrefractile crystals. With a first-order compensator, calcium pyrophosphate shows a faint blue against a red background when the axis of the crystal is parallel to the compensator.

The treatment of acute gout is safe and efficacious. Colchicine is the least expensive treatment but is associated with a high incidence of gastrointestinal side effects and should be used with great care. Indomethacin (25 mg every 4 to 6 hours with food or milk) is equally effective. During the symptom-free interval, specific treatment depends on a number of variables discussed briefly in Chapter 8. Acute pseudogout may be treated with similar agents, but the response is more rapid with joint aspiration and installation of corticosteroids.

Metatarsalgia

Metatarsalgia is pain of the metatarsal heads. It is rare in children and adolescents, and when present is frequently related to trauma or to osteochondritis of the second metatarsal head (Freiberg's disease). The latter condition is seen from ages 13 to 60, but is usually present in adolescents. The condition is diagnosed by x-ray, which shows squaring of the second metatarsal head. Other causes of metatarsalgia are summarized in Table 3–10.

When the transverse arch becomes depressed, the middle metatarsal heads bear a disproportionate amount of the weight. Symptoms consist of pain on weight bearing, and the examination shows tenderness over the metatarsal heads with formation of bunions and calluses. When there is no local tenderness, nerve entrapment or vascular causes should be sought. Metatarsalgia occurs commonly in old age, where the normal thickness of fat between the metatarsal head and the plantar surface is lost, and also in inflammatory arthritis of the joints. Treatment of painful metatarsal heads is directed towards treating any inflammatory process, as well as reducing pressure on the heads by a metatarsal pad *behind* the heads, by using a Thomas heel (to carry the medial counter forward to give a more anterior pivot point and to help supinate the foot during walking). These appliances should be prescribed with the exercises described below (Table 3–12).

HEEL PAIN

Pain of the heel is usually caused by plantar fasciitis with or without a "calcaneal spur." The diagnosis is made by physical examination alone, which shows joint tenderness at the anterior medial area of the calcaneus. An x-ray of the heel gives little or no additional information, as a heel spur is found as frequently in asymptomatic individuals and never changes the management. Calcaneal spurs seen in the spondylo-arthropathies are thought to have a distinctive x-ray appearance but the management of the heel pain is unchanged. The pain may arise from bursitis under the plantar fascial attachment to the periositis or tearing of the fibrous attachments to bone. When the pain is diffusely located over the heel pad, the diagnosis of painful heel pad is made, but the label should not make one think that the etiology is any better understood. In any case, resting the heel by whatever means possible will bring relief. Altering weight-bearing pressure can be accomplished by raising the heel one-quarter of an inch or by placing a doughnut under the heel, using a plastic heel cup, or by putting a hole in the sole of the shoe.

An occasional patient is so uncomfortable and unable to function that an injection of corticosteroids and Xylocaine into the area of the maximal tenderness from either the medial or lateral approach should be tried. Injections through the heel pad itself are more painful and are difficult to do because of the thick skin, but the localization of the injection is better. A rare patient is not helped by any of the above measures, and tenotomy of the plantar fascia at its posterior attachment may be suggested. The results are quite variable; no studies are available to offer criteria for patient selection.

Tendinitis and Bursitis

Three clinically significant but indistinguishable burase or tendonous insertion areas exist around the heel: the area around the Achilles tendon insertion, the postcalcaneal bursa, and the retrocalcaneal bursa. Repeated trauma to these areas may cause inflammation and pain. Paratendinitis occurs in runners, dancers, and jumpers or women who wear ill-fitting shoes ("pump bumps"). The area near the insertion may appear normal or may be swollen or have an audible or palpable rub with motion. Squeezing the tendon hurts.

Bursitis causes tenderness in an area less than a dime and may rarely have a visible inflamed lump. The treatment of tendinitis is joint rest. The more complete the rest the better, and a patient with a persistent problem should be totally immobilized with a cast. Local injections of steroids and/or Xylocaine are effective in other forms of bursitis and tendinitis but should not be done for Achilles tendon lesions since there is no tendon sheath and it is prone to rupture.

Achilles Tendon Rupture

A partial or complete tear of the Achilles tendon occurs in an area that is relatively avascular approximately 2″ above its point of insertion. Occurring typically in men between the ages of 40 and 50 years, tendon rupture is apt to occur with activities that place additional stress on a fully extended tendon, forceful ankle dorsiflexion to an unprepared ankle, or direct trauma to a taut tendon. Most tears are complete and partial tears usually become complete later on.

Walking and rising on one's toes are impossible with a complete tear. The major complaint is pain in the lower calf and heel. With a complete tear, a palpable gap may be felt as the gastrocnemius is retracted. With the patient prone, squeezing the calf does not move the ankle because plantar flexion cannot occur.

Tendon tears must be surgically repaired as soon as possible. Delay beyond 2 months decreases the chance of a successful result. Referral is needed at the time of diagnosis.

Calcaneal Apophysitis (Sever's Disease)

Children with heel pain are most likely to have osteochondritis of the posterior apophysis of the heel. The pain is below the attachment of the Achilles tendon, is frequently bilateral, and is aggravated by running or standing on tiptoes. Walking may be symptom free and the only complaint may be sensitivity to touch or pressure. X-rays are usually of no help, though occasionally there is unilateral fragmentation with bony condensation of the epiphysis.

The condition is self-limited and, thus, the treatment is solely symptomatic. A built-up heel lessens the pull of the Achilles tendon. Joint immobilization or a crutch are also helpful.

Subtalar Arthritis

Arthritis of the subtalar joint may refer to the heel and, thus, if a person complains of heel pain and there is no tenderness about the abovementioned structures, the subtalar joint must be examined. The treatment depends on the specific form of arthritis, but symptomatic treatment can be offered with a heel cup or a rigid posterior splint. If joint rest is unsatisfactory, surgical fusion may be indicated.

ANKLE PAIN

Sprained Ankle

The sprained ankle is the most common injury of the lower extremity. It may be a simple strain of the ligaments or a tearing of the ligaments with or without avulsion of the bones to which they are attached. The most severe injury, fracture dislocation, is obvious and requires an orthopedic surgeon. As with other traumatic injuries around joints, tears of ligaments and fractures must be diagnosed early so that prompt treatment can be instituted and disability prevented.

The major ligaments of the ankle joint are the lateral and medial collateral ligaments, which stabilize the ankle. The medial ligaments are taut in the neutral position, but the posterior strands are lax in plantar flexion and the anterior fibers are relaxed in dorsiflexion. The lateral collateral ligaments remain taut in all ranges of plantar flexion. When the foot is in plantar flexion, an unstable position, the ankle is most vulnerable to injury. The most common sprain occurs from inversion stress with the foot in plantar flexion and results in stretching of the lateral collateral anterior talofibular ligaments. If inversion stress occurs with the foot in neutral position, the calcaneofibular ligaments receives the stretch force. Eversion strains are less common and are more likely to be associated with a fracture.

After inspection and palpation, place the foot in plantar flexion and invert gently. Pain with this maneuver points to lateral ligamentous structures. Next, move the foot into dorsiflexion and invert; with inversion strain, pain should be considerably diminished. If the foot is placed in plantar flexion and everted, the medial ligaments are stressed. To minimize discomfort, move the ankle slowly. Tenderness over a ligament is a helpful sign if the patient is not uncomfortable with minimal palpation. Palpate the medial and lateral malleoli to check for a malleolar fracture or a tibiofibular ligament tear. Severe pain on motion with point tenderness directly over the malleolus is more indicative of fracture than sprain.

If there is significant soft-tissue swelling, a careful examination and stress x-ray views of the ankle are essential for proper diagnosis. In a simple strain, the talus remains in its proper position and no gap may be palpated between it and the malleolus during passive inversion of the ankle. Early on, protective muscle spasm may limit movement and deceive the physician into thinking that the joint is stable when it is not. Therefore, any *severe* sprain by history should be treated as a potential tear until x-rays are performed.

All significant ankle injuries (i.e., impressive trauma history, severe soft-tissue swelling, audible "snap," sensation of "tearing") need to be x-rayed with manipulation to look for tilting of the talus within the mortice, a sign of a ligament tear.

Eversion Sprains

Because of the strength of the deltoid ligaments, eversion stress is more likely to result in a fracture than a sprain. A sprain of the medial ligaments may tear the inferior tibiofibular ligament and cause the ankle mortice to widen and lead to an unstable ankle joint.

On radiological examination, the pathognomonic sign is widening of the joint space between the medial border of the talus and medial malleolus. The aim of treating a torn deltoid and an inferior tibiofibular ligament is to approximate the two malloli in order to reform the mortice so that the talus may rest snugly. Whether this should be done by casting or internal fixation is controversial.

Treatment

Because hemorrhage and fluid distend the joint capsule and stretch ligaments, immediate treatment is directed at controlling swelling. Swelling can be minimized by a) a firm but nonconstricting elastic bandage of the foot to mid-lower leg, b) ice for the first day, and c) elevation of the leg. Analgesics have been discussed in a previous section.

If only a strain is diagnosed, elastic bandaging should be done for 7 to 10 days with ice packs for the first day. *Passive* non-weight-bearing range-of-motion exercises of the foot should be started after the acute pain has subsided to maintain joint mobility and to prevent contractures of the Achilles tendon. When swelling has subsided or disappeared, and reexamination confirms that no ligament has been torn, the ankle should be taped for several weeks.

Severe sprains with avulsion or ligamentous tears are treated by casting or surgical repair of completely avulsed ligaments and all should be referred.

FLAT FEET

Flat feet are common; symptoms from flat feet are not. Many persons with complete flat feet have no trouble, while others are practically disabled. African Americans commonly have severely pronated feet with complete flattening of the longitudinal arch and a hallux valgus without any symptoms. In normal infants, the fat pad under the longitudinal arch, tibial torsion, and ligamentous laxity combine to give the appearance of flat feet. No treatment is needed: Infants develop an arch around 2 to 3 years of age. The majority of flat feet are "relaxed" flat feet, which can easily be recognized clinically as feet with a good longitudinal arch that disappears on weight bearing and reforms when the patient stands on the toes. Treatment is almost never required.

A classification of flat feet is given in Table 3–11. Approximately 1% of flat feet are rigid flat feet. The rigid flat foot is a pronated foot with an inflexible, depressed arch with soft-tissue contracture. Although rigid flat feet are rare and treatment is difficult and controversial, it is important to recognize and refer congenital cases of rigid flat feet. Paralytic flat feet should be referred and are not discussed.

Supple or flexible flat feet are easily manipulated to look like normal feet. A patient with supple flat feet may have lax ligaments, but generalized hypermobility, which requires that evidence of hypermobility be found at three different joints, is unusual.

TABLE 3–11. CLASSIFICATION OF FLAT FOOT DEFORMITY

I.	Flexible
II.	Rigid
	Tarsal coalition
	Arthrosis of the subtalar joint
	Congenital convex pes valgus or vertical talus
III.	Paralytic
	Cerebral palsy
	Miscellaneous (including poliomyelitis)

Flexible Flat Feet

Patients with mild deformity rarely present with symptoms, and there is no evidence that mild deformity will lead to symptoms later in life or that the treatment will increase the height of the arch.

Likewise, it is rare for patients with moderate deformity to have foot or leg symptoms. The often-mentioned symptoms of easy foot fatigue, discomfort in the arch, and calf pain are uncommonly encountered. Some physicians believe that this deformity is not self-correcting and that symptoms may develop as a result of degenerative changes in the tarsal joints. There is no evidence that the conventional treatment for moderate deformity (arch support, inner heel wedge, and an extended heel counter on the medial side of the shoe) affect a lasting change. Corrective shoes for growing children are expensive and a child may frustrate the "therapy" by preferring to walk without shoes.

Moderate to severely deformed flat feet may present with symptoms of foot pain. The symptoms are usually related to tight heel cords or to a painful callus under the head of the talus and/or degenerative arthritis at the tarsal joint. Conservative therapy is usually pursued, although whether the long-term outcome is altered is unanswered. In one short-term study, the use of a plastic heel mold in ten children with flexible flat feet showed in a 2-year follow-up: a) elimination of local pain in the anterior tibial muscles and diffuse pain in 6 out of 10 subjects who had prior complaints to the study and b) 8 out of 10 subjects showed improvement in gait as demonstrated by more even shoe wear. However, in patients with relatively fixed foot deformities, the inserts did not achieve lasting structural changes after the 2-year wear period was complete. Surgical approaches to supple, flat feet are numerous and unproven.

Treatment of flexible flat feet

Pain is the primary indication for treatment. If the feet are painful along the longitudinal arch or inner border, or if there is pain in the calves and the anterior tibial muscle, conservative treatment can be beneficial. If pain is present

TABLE 3–12. EXERCISES FOR PAINFUL FLAT FEET

1. *Frequency.* Graduate up to five repetitions twice a day.

2. *Foot Exercises*
   A. Flex toes
   B. Stand with toes turned inward and roll on side of foot
   C. Pick up small marbles with toes
   D. Rising up and down on toes
   E. Walk increasing distances daily

3. *Stretching Exercises*
   A. Sit squarely, roll feet outward until soles are nearly parallel, relax (pronators)
   B. Stand facing two feet from a wall, swing towards the wall keeping heels on floor and knees locked

at rest, weight bearing should be discouraged until the acute episode is over. Strengthening exercises of the plantar flexors and adductors, and stretching of the dorsiflexors and pronators are outlined in Table 3–12.

Many individuals will benefit from a longitudinal arch pad of felt, cork, or rubber, and a heel wedge just beneath the sole. Properly made supports are comfortable, support the arch, and favor walking on the outer rather than the inner border of the foot. About one-half of arch supports used are manufactured in a small number of standard sizes. While these can be obtained readily, they may not fit precisely and do not give as much relief as those that are made from plaster impressions from the patient's foot. In the uncomplicated cases, supports are usually worn for a number of months and then are gradually given up as normal strength and alignment return to the foot. In older patients and in refractory cases, permanent arch supports may be required.

Rigid Flat Foot

The rigid flat foot is a flat foot that cannot be passively corrected. In these conditions, some form of therapy is usually required, although some patients may never require treatment. Assessing the medial stability of the talus is essential in judging whether active treatment or referral is necessary. If a prominent head of the talus is palpated medially, suggesting insufficient talonavicular joint stability, or if there is a rigid calcaneovalgus position, permanent deformity is likely. The management strategy is specialized and requires consultation.

Congenital rigid flat feet with a vertical talus should be considered in any infant with a rigid calcaneovalgus foot that fails to correct in the first few months of life. Walking is not delayed, but when the child starts to stand, the deformity is worsened and the feet take on a "rocker-bottom" appearance with the midfoot resting on the ground, and the heel and forefoot suspended off the ground.

Congenital coalition is the second important cause of rigid flat feet due to congenital fusion of one or more tarsal bones. A foot with congenital fusion is rigidly flat and remains flat whether or not the patient is bearing weight. There is considerable limitation of inversion and eversion. It frequently results in secondary symptomatic strain or spasm of the peroneal and extensor muscles. The most frequent coalitions occur between the talus and calcaneus, and between the navicular and calcaneus, but other combinations are seen.

In general, persons with congenital coalition start to complain of foot pain during adolescence. Common symptoms are aching in the medial aspect of the foot and ankle, and pain in the lateral peroneal and calf region from muscle spasm. Approximately 10% of these patients with congenital coalition or peroneal spastic flat feet will be sufficiently symptomatic to require an operation, which is generally a triple arthrodesis.

PAINFUL FOOT, NORMAL EXAM

A painful foot without physical findings of joint or soft-tissue problems suggests peripheral vascular disease or an entrapment neuropathy.

Nerve Entrapment Syndromes of the Foot

A Morton's neuroma gives neuritic pain of the third and fourth toes or, less commonly, of the second and third toes. It is an entrapment of the interdigital nerve and it occurs most commonly in middle-aged women. Pain occurs with weight bearing and eventually at rest. Patients characteristically want to remove their shoes and massage their feet.

The examination confirms clinical suspicion. Pressure between the metatarsal heads or compression of the metatarsal heads reproduces the pain, whereas, common metatarsalgia is tender over the metatarsal heads. Numbness in the contiguous area of the toes or the neuroma itself may occasionally be found.

Treatment consists of supporting the transverse arch in a suitable broad shoe. Local injection of steroids often gives relief, but surgical excision of the neuroma is sometimes required.

The interdigital nerves may also be compressed by the transverse metatarsal ligament over which the nerves pass. This is particularly likely to occur if the toes are hyperextended at the metatarsal joints. The symptoms are similar to a Morton's neuroma. The treatment is preventing hyperextension of the toes by correcting occupational postures, proscribing high heels, and using a metatarsal bar.

Compression of the posterior tibial nerve or its plantar branches within the tunnel formed by the medial malleous and the ligament between the talus and the calcaneus (the tarsal tunnel) produces neurogenic pain of the lateral or medial plantar areas or the heel, depending on which branch is involved. The diagnosis is made by the history of burning pain in the distribution of the plantar nerve. Percussion of the tarsal tunnel just anterior to the mallelous reproduces the pain exactly. The toe flexors are weak, and there is intrinsic muscle wasting and sensory loss of the true plantar surface. Conservative treatment consists of injecting the tunnel with corticosteroids and correcting pronation of the foot.

Injury of the anterior tibial nerve (also called the deep peroneal) produces numbness in the first web space, weakness of first toe extension, and tenderness over the nerve as it becomes superficial below the cruciate ligament.

Footstrain

Acute footstrain is self-limited and subsides with rest. Chronic foot strain may arise if excessive stress is repeated or if normal stress is imposed upon a mechanical abnormality. Tender areas may be noted on the medial border of the plantar fascia. The posterior tibial ligament (under and behind the medial malleolus) and the second metatarsal head are also sites of pain. Treatment of foot strain is essentially the treatment of the adult flatfoot: first rest, then gradually increase exercise and arch support.

REFERENCES

Amis JA, Gangl PM: When inversion injury is more than a "sprained ankle." J Musculoskeletal Med 4:68–87, 1987.

Bergreld JA: Symposium management of acute ankle sprains. Contemp Orthop 13:83–114, 1986.

Cass JR, Morrey BF: Ankle instability — current concepts, diagnosis, and treatment. Mayo Clin Proc 59:165–170, 1984.

Clement DB, Taunton JR, Smart GW: Achilles tendinitis and peritendinitis: Etiology and treatment. Am J Sports Med 12:179–184, 1984.

Danielson L: Incidence of osteoarthritis of the hip (coxarthrosis). Clin Orthop 45:67–72, 1966.

De Lisa JA, Saueed MA: The tarsal tunnel syndrome. Muscle Nerve 6:664–670, 1983.

Feinstein PA: Orthopaedic management of the three general types of symptomatic flatfoot. Orthop Rev 8:123–129, 1979.

Fischer RL: Conservative treatment of patellofemoral pain. Orthop Clin North Am 17:269–272, 1986.

Gibson T, Burry HL, Poswillo P, Glass J: Effect of intra-articular corticosteroid injections on primate cartilage. Ann Rheum Dis 36:74–79, 1976.

Graham CE: Painful heel syndrome: Rationale of diagnosis and treatment. Foot Ankle 3:261–267, 1983.

Graham CE, Graham DM: Morton's neuroma: A microscopic evaluation. Foot Ankle 5:150–153, 1984.

Grossman RB, Nicholas JA: Common disorders of the knee. Orthop Clin North Am 8:619–623, 1977.

Jones RE, Smith EC, Reisch JS: Effects of medial meniscectomy in patients older than forty years. J Bone Joint Surg [Am] 60A:783–786, 1978.

Liang MH, Cullen K, Poss R. Primary total hip and knee replacement surgery. Evaluation of Patients. Ann Intern Med 97:735–739, 1982.

Liang MH, Fries JF: Asymptomatic hyperuricemia: The case for conservative management. Ann Intern Med 88:666–670, 1978.

Lloyd-Roberts GC: Osteoarthritis of the hip: A study of the clinical pathology. J Bone Joint Surg [Am] 37B:8–47, 1955.

MacEwen GD, Zembo MM: Current trends in the treatment of congenital dislocation of the hip. Orthopedics 10:1663–1669, 1987.

Maquet P: Mechanics and osteoarthritis of the patellofemoral joint. Clin Orthop 144:70–73, 1979.

Palumbo PM Jr: Dynamic patellar brace in patellofemoral disorders: A preliminary report. Am J Sports Med 9:45, 1981.

Rasmussen KJ, Fano N. Trochanteric bursitis: Treatment by corticosteroid injection. Scand J Rheum 14:417–420, 1985.

Roberts WN, Liang MH, Stern SH: Colchicine for acute gout: Assessment of risks and benefits. JAMA 257:1920–1922, 1987.

Scranton PE: Metatarsalgia: A clinical review of diagnosis and management. Foot and Ankle 1:229–234, 1981.

Soren A, Fetto JF: Pathology, clinic, and treatment of Osgood–Schlatter disease. *Orthopedics* 7:230–234, 1984.

Thompson FM, Hamilton WG: Problems of the second metatarsophalangeal joint. Orthopedics 10:83–89, 1987.

Vainionpaa S, Laike E, Kirves P, Tuisaner P: Tibial osteotomy for osteoarthritis of the knee. A five to ten year follow-up study. J Bone Joint Surg [Am] 63A:938–946, 1981.

Vegso JJ, Harmon LE: Nonoperative management of athletic ankle injuries. Clin Sport Med 1:85–98, 1982.

Zarins B, Adams M: Knee injuries in sports. N Engl J Med 318:950–961, 1988.

4 Low Back Pain

Low back pain is the most common musculoskeletal complaint seen in an ambulatory care setting. Though often thought of as an orthopedic problem, back complaints are the seventh most common problem seen by internists. Low back pain affects 80% of all persons at some time in their lives. Back pain is second only to the common cold in days of missed work — 93 million days a year in this country — and is the number one cause of activity restriction in people under 45.

Students of back pain identify a long list of conditions that may give rise to the symptom, but there is little information on the relative frequency of these causes in an unselected patient population, or whether, in fact, understanding the source of pain significantly changes the management strategy or ultimately the patient outcome. Identifying the precise anatomical source of pain is reassuring to the physician, but the basic therapeutic options are unchanged, except for specific entities that will be described in this chapter. The taxonomy includes vague "diagnoses" such as sciatica, lumbosacral strain, low back strain, lumbar intervertebral joint derangement, lumbago, etc. Other labels such as herniated disc, degenerative joint disease, and arthritis imply a more specific diagnosis, but the diagnostic criteria are not uniform.

ECOLOGY OF LOW BACK PAIN

In ambulatory patients, nine out of ten instances of low back pain are self-limited. Since diagnosis is based almost solely on clinical findings, the specific "cause" of low back pain depends on disease definitions and the setting. Table 4–1 gives the possible causes for low back pain in ambulatory adults.

Many persons with low back pain treat themselves with time and simple home remedies. Of those who go to a physician with acute low back pain, 44% are better within a week and 92% within a month, and only 8% have pain persisting more than 2 months. Practices with a greater percentage of older

TABLE 4–1. CAUSES OF LOW BACK PAIN IN THE AMBULATORY SETTING

Strain or unknown	93.2%
Herniated disc	6
Tauma	.2
Ankylosing spondylitis and neoplasm	.5
Other	.8

patients, compensation cases, and laborers may not experience such good outcomes. When low back pain is due to disc protrusions with evidence of radiculopathy, pain is progressively improved by 6 weeks, the sensory examination is improved by 6 months, and reflexes may or may not change. With the exception of progressive neuromotor symptoms, the initial treatment of nearly all causes of low back pain is conservative: analgesics and/or anti-inflammatory agents, bed rest, and patient education.

DIAGNOSTIC STRATEGY

The practical task for the generalist is to sort out the benign and self-limited cases of back pain from the serious cases and to recognize when the pain is a symptom of other problems. X-ray examinations of the lumbosacral spine, the major expense in a reflexive approach to the diagnosis of low back pain, are insensitive. Many spinal lesions including disease of the disc that may cause back pain are not detected by radiology. X-ray findings of osteophytes, narrowed disc space, lumbarization, sacralization, mild scoliosis, facet arthrosis, subluxation, and spina bifida occulta are found equally in symptomatic and asymptomatic backs.

When the history and physical examination are compatible with a benign, self-limited disease, x-rays have limited clinical utility. X-rays are indicated in the following situations:

1. Unimproved or worsening symptoms; symptoms longer than a month with treatment
2. New onset of back pain without antecedent trauma under age 15 or over 50
3. Back pain after significant trauma (direct blow to spine, fall on buttock, car accident)
4. Severe back pain
5. History or physical examination suggestive of sacroiliitis
6. Pain not significantly relieved by bed rest
7. Previous vertebral fracture, surgery
8. Anxious person who will not be reassured by clinical examination alone
9. Spinal deformity or mass
10. Known malignancy
11. Constitutional symptoms (fever, weight lost)

A radiologic examination of the back includes anteroposterior, lateral, and coned-down view of S5–L1. Oblique views contribute little additional information. Forward and extension films are needed to detect displacement of the bony structures such as in spondylolisthesis. Electroneuromyography documents radiculopathy and measures nerve conduction loss. If a nerve root is compressed, the earliest clinical signs are loss or diminution of deep tendon reflexes. After several weeks of compression, sometimes six, objective muscle wasting or a decrease in strength is noticed. The electroneuromyogram is helpful in establishing the baseline, measuring change, as well as ascertaining whether the denervation is acute or chronic. For most cases, if surgical intervention is not a possibility, the electroneuromyogram may not provide information beyond that of the examination and the patient's symptoms. Myelograms should be done in persons with low back pain only if surgery is contemplated.

In evaluation of low back pain, the primary physician must distinguish between four groups of conditions (Table 4–2)

1. Low back pain from mechanical problems, with or without nerve-root compression
2. Back pain from lesions of the bone
3. Inflammatory back pain
4. Psychological back pain

These clinical groups direct the evaluation strategy and treatment program.

Practically, the problem is to separate those patients with mechanical causes from all the others in the first visit and do not miss causes of back pain that require prompt treatment.

These are: (mnemonic = *MAIDS*)

1. *M*yelitis
2. *A*bdominal catastrophe: perforated viscus, abdominal aneurysm
3. *I*nfection (spine, disc, epidural space)
4. Herniated *D*isc, with important or progressive neurological involvement
5. *S*pinal cord compression (tumor, disc)

Atypical clinical features (red flags — Table 4–3) suggest diagnoses other than mechanical causes. If the history and physical examination are typical of a mechanical origin, conservative treatment is indicated. The patient should be followed to ensure adequate pain control and should be seen again in 3 weeks to ensure resolution of the problem and to reinforce back care instructions and specific exercise therapy. The salient history, a short fail-safe examination for acute low back pain, and detailed examination for problematic back pain follow.

OFFICE EVALUATION OF LOW BACK PAIN

The Back Pain History

The complaint of pain in the back may mean discomfort anywhere from the base of the neck to the buttocks. Thus, the individual should be asked to point to the

TABLE 4–2. TYPES OF BACK PAIN

Mechanical
Intrinsic
Chronic postural strain
Severe scoliosis
Spondylolysis
Leg-length discrepancy
Transitional vertebrae
Degenerative
Herniated disc
Osteoarthritis
Trauma
Lumbar strain — acute and chronic
Fracture of vertebral body or transverse process, spondylolisthesis
Subluxated facet joint
Osseous
Tumor
Benign — hemangiomas, bone cyst, meningioma, dermoid, etc.
Malignant — metastatic and primary (neural, multiple myeloma, chordoma)
Metabolic bone disease
Osteoporosis — fracture
Osteomalacia
Hyperparathyroidism with osteitis fibrosa cystica
Inflammatory
Soft tissue
Tendinitis
Fibrositis
Bursitis
Arthritis
Ankylosing spondylitis
Rheumatoid arthritis
Sacroiliitis
Infection
Acute — disc, sacroiliac, or bone
Chronic — tuberculosis, fungal, chronic osteomyelitis
Psychological
Functional
Malingering

offending area and to where it radiates or spreads. Referred pain is rarely felt below the knee, whereas pain due to root irritation radiates to the calf and foot. An L5 root radiates down the front of the thigh. A good history of the onset, duration, and tempo of the symptoms suggests the diagnostic possibilities. If the pain started suddenly, it is likely to be a tear of the muscles, ligaments, or disc, or a fracture. If the pain started gradually and is chronic or subacute, chronic low back pain, tumor, metabolic bone disease, or spondylitis are possibilities. The sudden onset of pain following activity suggests a mechanical basis for the symptoms. Biomechanical pain is worst at the end of the day and is vaguely described and localized. Is the pain getting worse? Is it because the attacks are more frequent, more severe, and more prolonged, or is it because the patient has lost his tolerance and is fed up with the symptom?

TABLE 4–3. LOW BACK PAIN — (RED FLAGS)

Clinical Data	Diagnostic Significance
Pain not relieved by supine position with hips flexed	Infection, osseous lession, spondylitis, ? compliance
Pain worse with walking	Spinal stenosis
Pain worse with hyperextension of the spine and improved by flexing the spine	
Pain (stiffness) worse in morning	Spondylitis, epiphysitis
Acute, severe pain without precipitants	Abdominal aneurysm, compression fracture, spinal vascular accident, ruptured viscus, herniated disc
Pain increased by cough, sneeze, or Valsalva	Nerve-root compression
Pain described as numbness, stinging, tingling	Nerve-root compression
Systemic symptoms	Infection, tumor
Other joints symptomatic	Inflammatory arthritis
Pain > 1 month	Metabolic bone disease, herniated disc compensation, psychological, structural, tumor
Bilateral radiation	Tumor, central herniation, spondylitis
Onset < 30 years old or > 50	Tumor, metabolic disease, epiphysitis
Fever	Infection
Synovitis	Inflammatory arthritis
Midline deformities	Structural defect, tumor
(palpable step, midline hair)	(dermoid, epidermoid)
Neuromotor deficit or asymmetry	Nerve-root compression
Progressive neuromotor deficit	Central herniation
Bilateral neurological deficits	Space occupying lesion of spinal canal, spinal vascular accident
Multiple nerve-root involvement	
Nerve-root level above L1	
Positive Babinski's, Clonus	Myelopathy
Inconsistent examination	Psychogenic
Flat or theatrical affect	Psychogenic

TABLE 4–4. PREDICTING LOCATION OF LESION BY EXAM

Nerve Root (Level)	Pain	Sensory Deficit	Weakness	Reflex Loss
L4 (L3–L4)	Lower back, posterolateral thigh	Anteromedial thigh	Quadriceps	Patellar
L5 (L4–L5)	Low back, hip lateral thigh and leg	Outer edge of calf and great toe	Dorsiflexors of great toe and ankle	None
S1 (L5–S1)	Back of thigh, outer calf to foot and lateral toes	Outer calf and foot and lesser toes	Plantar flexion	Achilles

Disc disease occurs usually between L3 and S1 (Table 4–4) and is unilateral. When pain originates above the L3 level or is bilateral, infection, tumor, or spondylitis should be considered. When biomechanical causes of low back pain recur or flare, the pattern usually repeats itself. If the pattern is different or the pain is worsening, think tumor.

Nerve-root compression is suggested when pain comes on rapidly in the distribution of the sensory dermatome of that nerve root. Dorsal nerve-root pain is sharp, lancinating, and accompanied by paresthesias and numbness. Paresthesias or numbness felt over the lateral border of the foot suggest an S1 lesion; and over the dorsal of the foot, an L5 lesion. Increasing tension on the nerve roots by coughing, sneezing, or straining while defecating can exacerbate the pain. In contrast, pain in deep structures such as ligaments, fascia, muscles, and periosteum are vaguely localized, aching in character, radiate widely, and are generally slow in onset and long in duration.

What activities make the pain worse or better? Mechanical pain arising from elements of the spine is almost always aggravated by movement and relieved by rest. Pain referred to the back from the gastrointestinal tract, female reproductive system, and solid organs in the abdomen are unaltered by spinal movement. An occasional person with disc disease finds the pain worse in bed, but he or she may actually be sleeping prone, hyperextending their spine and exacerbating the pain. Inflammatory back pain, ankylosing spondylitis, and Scheuermann's disease (epiphysitis of the dorsal vertebrae), in contrast, cause pain or stiffness that is worse after resting and is improved by activity.

In an emotionally well person, pain out of proportion to physical findings for which the person cannot find a comfortable position suggests an infected disc (discitis) or an epidural abscess. Pain is subject to a host of environmental and psychological factors, but pain that interferes with work, recreation, or sleep, or that occurs in a person who "never has pain" is important.

Most persons are concerned not only about the cause of their symptoms but also about their significance. Is it cancer? Is it arthritis? To many persons, arthritis calls forth a relentless disease leading eventually to crippling and dependency. Such feats are common and are frequently unexpressed. The physician must explain the pathogenesis of back symptoms and what the symptoms are not.

In individuals prone to fretting, the anxiety about their symptoms may be more disabling than the pain itself. Reasonable concern becomes pathological worry. No amount of reassurance seems to be sufficient. These individuals confuse hurt with harm and believe that any activity that hurts the back will lead to irreparable damage.

In some persons, the back pain complaint is a camouflage for depression or an excuse for inability to cope. Therapeutic measures directed at the organic lesion alone will not work: Treatment must be directed at the patient as a whole.

For a manual worker in a strenuous job, recurrent back pain can be a disaster financially if it prevents the patient from being employable, and the symptoms may be exaggerated far out of proportion to the actual organic problem. Likewise, the continued necessity to claim disability for disability benefits or workmen's compensation may make continued back pain an economic "necessity."

Examination for Acute Back Pain

Acute back pain is back pain of less than a week's duration with no recent history of back symptoms. The examination for acute low back pain should be done in an orderly way; a cursory examination is worse than no examination at all. Ask to observe the patient while he or she undresses to note abnormal or painful movements. Exaggerated lordosis or flattening of the normal lordosis should be noted. The latter is seen in anklylosing spondylitis and with muscle spasm. Lumbar lordosis is increased in pregnancy or obesity to keep the body's center of gravity above the feet.

With the patient standing with the feet about a foot apart, inspect the back for a pelvic tilt that may be due to a leg-length discrepancy, scoliosis, or muscle spasm. Note the presence of scoliosis. Fixed scoliosis due to structural problems differs from secondary scoliosis due to muscle spasm, painful splinting, and leg-length discrepancy, which disappears on recumbency. Spasm of the sacrospinalis muscles or gluteii will make these muscles more prominent when compared with the normal side. A midline dimple or tufts of hair (Faun's beard) indicate a pilonidal cyst, spina bifida occulta, or a dermoid.

The range and rhythm of spinal movements should be tested. In forward flexion, the normal lumbar lordosis flattens and flexes until the spine is a smooth curve from the sacrum to the occiput. Foward bending assesses the mobility of the back, the hamstrings, and the hips. Functional or nonstructural scoliosis disappears on flexion, whereas structural scoliosis is exaggerated on bending. A prolapsed intervertebral disc with nerve-root irritation results in marked limitation of forward flexion without lumbar movement. Such persons will frequently show deviation of the trunk toward the painful side on forward flexion, but extension and rotation are relatively smooth and symmetrical. In spondylolisthesis, an abnormal step in the lower lumbar spine may be palpated, which disappears in flexion.

With the individual standing, the strength of the gastrocnemius is tested by having the patient stand on tip toe. Fatigability or asymmetric rising suggests a lesion of the S1 nerve root or weak quadriceps. The dorsiflexors of the ankle are assessed by having the person walk on the heels; difficulty with this maneuver points to an L5 nerve root. Peroneal nerve damage may also cause impaired heel walk; if there is difficulty, check the strength of eversion of the foot, which is solely a peroneal nerve function. Some persons with sciatica will have pain when the ankle dorsiflexors are used with the knee extended and give the impression of weakness when none exists.

Sensation is checked in the sitting position. Areas of sensory innervation are variable. Testing the autonomous areas is an efficient way to elicit hypesthesia. The S1 root innervates the sole and lateral border of the foot, and its autonomous area is the area just behind the lateral malleolus and the bottom of the little toe. The L5 root receives sensation from the dorsum foot and the anterior aspect of the lower leg, and its autonomous area is the first interdigital space and the lateral calf below the level of the patella. The L4 nerve root innervates the anteromedial thigh, and its autonomous sensory zone is a triangle with the apex over the patella and the base above the patella. When sensory and motor signs conflict, make the diagnosis based on the more reliable motor signs rather than the sensory deficits.

Stretching of the nerve roots (straight leg raising) may be done sitting. The patient is instructed to sit with the legs dangling over the side of the bed. One leg is fixed by the examiner and the affected limb is extended passively at the knee. In sciatica, no resistance or pain is noted until the lumbar lordosis is flattened (when the knee has extended 45°), at which point the patient compensates by leaning backward, frequently grabbing on to the table to prevent lurching backward. In sciatica, the individual is unable to sit erect with both knees extended. He or she must either flex the knee of the affected extremity or lean backward to avoid the pain associated with nerve-root stretching. When no sciatica exists, the patient has no difficulty in sitting erect with the affected knee fully extended.

In summary, a screening back examination is done simply by the following maneuvers. The person is observed walking, undressing, and getting up on the examination table. The motion of the spine in forward flexion and lateral bending is checked. The person is instructed to walk forward on the heels and then the toes to screen for muscle weakness. A check of the deep tendon reflexes, a sensory examination of the autonomous sensory zones, and sciatic nerve stretch are done with the patient sitting. Finally, the hips are checked for internal and external rotation. If there is any evidence of sacral nerve-root compression, the anal sphincteric reflex should be sought.

Examination for Chronic Low Back Pain

Chronic low back pain is back pain of greater than a month's duration. A screening examination should be done, but an additional history must be taken and extra maneuvers are done to look for unusual causes of low back pain. The goal of the physical examination is to reproduce the pain during the examination. Reproduction of the pain by a specific maneuver usually yields a stronger diagnostic conclusion than reproduction by palpation alone.

First, the patient is observed as he or she walks and sits down. In the sitting position, differences in the thigh and calf muscle circumferences provide subtle evidence for a neurological deficit. Normally, up to a half inch (13 mm) increase in thigh circumference may occur on the dominant side. Some persons have mixed dominance, using their right hand for writing but their left foot for kicking. If the dominant foot has a lesser circumference than the other side, significant atrophy is certain on the dominant side. Muscle strength, straight leg raising, and peripheral pulses and reflexes are checked in the sitting position as well.

During the strength exam the ankle dorsiflexors are checked with the knee flexed. Lesions of the fifth lumbar root may cause weakness of the extensor hallicus longus before any weakness of the ankle dorsiflexors is clinically apparent. Similarly, S1 lesions may give rise to flexor hallicus longus weakness ("scrunch or claw your toes") before gastrocneumius weakness is demonstrable. Quadricep weakness may be demonstrated with the examiner resisting extension of the knee with the person supine and with the hips slightly flexed. Diffuse muscle weakness, jerky relaxation against resistance, or the ability to resist force in a fixed position but an inability to initiate movement against resistance is functional weakness. Diffuse muscle tenderness indicates inflammed muscles or nerve-root irritation. First sacral root irritation may be associated with calf tenderness; fifth lumbar root irritation with anterior tibial muscle tenderness; and fourth lumbar root irritation with quadriceps tenderness.

Muscle tenderness that may be either local or referred is often misattributed to spasm. True muscle spasm is present if there is a list that persists when the patient bends forward and if the scoliosis disappears in the sitting position. If bending to the right or left produces motion at different levels on one side compared to the other, muscle spasm is present. In the prone position, the paravertebral musculature is normally relaxed and the presence of localized, taut, tender muscles suggests true spasm.

Reproduction of the pain by a maneuver is the central goal in the physical examination. Straight leg raising in the supine position is the classic Laseque test for nerve-root irritation. The leg should be raised slowly, because the rest of the examination will be sabotaged if the pain produced is severe or unexpected. Pain on straight leg raising may be caused by sciatica or any painful lesion associated with a hamstring spasm. In patients with a central disc protrusion, straight leg raising induces mainly back pain. In patients with an intermediate protrusion with the herniated disc lying in contact with both the dura and the nerve root, back and leg pain predominate. Eighty percent of patients with lateral protrusion experience pain only in the leg.

Reproduction or aggravation of sciatic pain by dorsiflexion of the ankle at the limit of straight leg raising relieved by bending the knees is diagnostic of nerve-root irriation. If the knee is bent at the point where pain is relieved and the pressure is applied in the popliteal fossa over the sciatic nerve, pain in the back or down the leg is similarly diagnostic of a nerve-root lesion (bowstring sign). Straight leg raising of the symptom-free side that gives rise to pain in the affected side is virtually diagnostic of nerve-root compression as well.

If a person has back pain after the knee has been flexed and if the pain is worse on further flexion of the hip, a significant emotional component or hip disease is suspected. Malingerers and patients with chronic low back may learn that dorsiflexion of the ankle is supposed to cause pain. With the knee flexed 90°, the ankle can be dorsiflexed painlessly without stretching the sciatic nerve, except in malingerers.

In lesions involving the third and fourth lumbar roots, the patient will experience pain on stretching the femoral nerve. This test is performed with the patient lying face down. The hip is then extended, with the knee maintained in a slightly flexed position. This test is positive, indicating a lesion, if the patient experiences pain radiating down the front of the thigh. Back pain alone from hyperextension of the back is not of diagnostic significance, but when the maneuver causes pain radiating into both buttocks, spinal stenosis is likely.

Hip flexion contractures associated with tight hamstrings are common in persons with chronic low back pain. The individual with tight hamstrings stands with the knees and hips flexed to relieve the pull on his hamstrings, which results in a hip flexion contracture and an accentuated lumbar lordosis. Bilateral iliopsoas contractures lead to exaggerated lumbar lordosis, which predisposes individuals to chronic backache.

Impaired internal and external rotation of the hips may cause back pain at T12–L1, because if the individual is unable to rotate at the hips, he or she must rotate elsewhere. Always assess hip motion fully in a back examination. Because of the configuration of the femoral head, the hip may have a normal range of motion in flexion and may still have a loss of motion in extension, which can only be assessed with the individual prone.

Specific lateral tenderness in a triangle formed by the L5 and S1 spinous processes and the iliac crest points to injury of the iliolumbar ligament. Tenderness over the posterosuperior iliac spine at the insertion of the lumbodorsal fascia indicates injury to the fascial attachments. Pain in the sciatic notch suggests irritation of the nerve root. Pain medial to the sciatic notch over the ischial prominence suggests ischial bursitis.

In patients with chronic painful back pain, there may be a problem of distinguishing whether symptoms come from an organic or psychological cause. Operationally, it is best to assume that persons with chronic pain have both a somatic and a psychological component to their symptoms. Deliberate feigning of an illness or malingering is relatively rare compared with subconscious modulation of emotional factors or conversion of emotional problems to organic symptoms.

Think of psychological factors when:

1. The appearance of comfort is out of proportion to the complaints of pain.
2. Pain is described dramatically.
3. Pain is localized to a nonanatomical distribution.
4. Physical findings are inconsistent or variable.
   a. Pain on straight leg raising is not relieved by flexion of the knee and is aggravated by further flexion of the hip with the knee flexed.
   b. Inability to increase the range of flexion of the lumbar spine, even when kneeling on a chair. When the patient is kneeling, the hamstrings and sciatic nerves are relaxed, and the patient should be able to bend forward with a fair degree of comfort, even in the presence of marked root tension. Exceptions to the rule are patients with vertebral osteomyelitis, ankylosing spondylitis, or massive herniations of the disc.
   c. Positive Hoover's test. With the patient lying, the "weak" leg cannot be lifted off the table, and no pressure is exerted down by the contralateral heel, which is cupped by the examiner's hand.
5. Secondary gain is present. Financial gain or the ability to manipulate the environment for attention, affection, or work avoidance.
6. The system's review is a litany of complaints.
7. Cog-wheel weakness
8. Sudden jerks with complaints of pain during the examination. Such a jerk would normally aggravate the pain and is a histrionic response.

In patients with chronic pain, additional evaluation directed towards understanding the patient's perception of the symptoms is necessary. Does the patient understand why he or she has pain, its probable prognosis, the prescribed therapies? What does the patient expect from this evaluation? Does the pain interfere with the person's normal activities? Does the patient want treatment, or does he or she want reassurance that nothing is serious and that it will go away? How do other family members or friends respond to the pain?

In summary, on the basis of a history directed at eliciting the precipitants, the quality and the modifying factors of the back pain, and an examination that specifically seeks neuromuscular involvement, abnormalities of the spine, and focal tenderness, the physician can confidently sort persons who present with back pain into five diagnostic groups:

- Mechanical back pain
- Bone lesions
- Inflammatory back pain
- Referred back pain
- Psychogenic

Do not miss the MAIDS conditions on the initial visit. These latter conditions should be suspected whenever there are red flags or atypical features of the case. The major diagnostic groups and their treatment are discussed in the sections that follow.

MECHANICAL AND STRUCTURAL CAUSES OF BACK PAIN

Disc Disease

Since the work of Mixter and Barr, the central importance of the intervertebral disc in the pathogenesis of low back pain has been recognized. Thus it is important to understand its biology and how it may produce back symptoms.

All individuals eventually will have degenerative changes of the disc. By age 20 to 30, maximum development of the disc has occurred, and the water content is maximal, approximating 80%. Thereafter, fragmentation of the annulus occurs. Later the cartilage plates become thin and fissured, with a progressive decrease in water content, mucopolysaccharides, and proteoglycans. With these changes, the disc has a decreased ability to maintain the normally high intradiscal pressure, which buffers vertical forces on the spine, thus making the spinal structures more susceptible to trauma.

The evidence implicating the intervertebral disc in the pathogenesis of some low back pain is:

1. Disc herniation is usually preceded by one or more attacks of low back pain.
2. Hypertonic saline or contrast media injected in the intradiscal space reproduces low back pain consistently.
3. Sutures have been placed on a variety of structures in and near the spine during back surgery. Preoperative pain is only reproduced by pulling on the nerve root, dorsal longitudinal ligament, and posterior annulus.

4. Nerve fibers exist only in the posterior part of the annulus of the intervertebral disc where ruptures commonly occur.

When the height of the intervertebral disc space is reduced by disc degeneration, disc removal, tears, or ruptures, the smooth roller action between the vertebral bodies is lost and movement becomes uneven. The resulting segmental hyperextension may stress the apophyseal (posterior) joints by excessive flexion, extension, and by backward and forward motion. Hyperextension of the spine is made worse if the patient has weak abdominal muscles, tight hamstrings, is overweight, is pregnant, or wears high heels.

Repeated damage of the posterior joints will lead to degenerative changes. This is true osteoarthritis of the spine. Gross lipping of the vertebral bodies, often referred to as osteoarthritis of the spine, is merely a manifestation of disc degeneration and may present without any changes in the posterior joints.

Disc Herniation

Acute disc protrusion occurs after trauma or degenerative changes in the disc. As a lumbar disc protrudes, the posterior longitudinal ligament containing pain-sensitive nerve endings is stretched. Protrusion through this ligament may also compress the lumbar nerve roots.

The most common sites for protrusion of the intervertebral disc are posterolaterally between the fourth and fifth lumbar vertebrae, compressing the fifth lumbar nerve, and between the fifth lumbar and first sacral vertebrae, compressing the first sacral root. When this occurs, the spinal nerve may be menaced as it passes through the intervertebral foramen. Intervertebral disc protrusion through the vertebral plate into the vertebral body gives rise to a Schmorl's nodule seen on x-rays.

A rare, but more serious protrusion is a central medial one, and if this occurs, the disc is completely extruded through the annulus fibrosis and the posterior longitudinal ligament, and compression of the cauda equina may occur. A midline disc protrusion is a surgical emergency and constitutes the only absolute indication for operation in lumbar disc protrusions. Involvement of the sacral nerves produces anesthesia of a saddle-shape distribution, bilateral leg weakness, absent ankle jerks, and sphincter disturbances. If pressure on the cauda equina is not relieved by laminectomy, the patient may be paralyzed.

Other Nerve Compression Syndromes

Any irritation or damage to nerves near the back may cause back pain. Sciatica can be caused by disc disease, an errantly place intramuscular injection, or by entrapment peripherally.

The pyriformis syndrome is thought to be caused by entrapment of the sciatic nerve as it passes in front of the pyriformis muscle and behind the obturator muscles where the sciatic nerve emerges from the pelvis at the exterior portion of the sciatic notch. Straight leg raising produces pain that is relieved by externally rotating the leg while it is still in the raised position. With internal rotation, the pyriformis is taut and compresses the sciatic nerve, while external rotation relaxes the muscle and reduces pressure on the nerve.

Bony compression of the emerging nerve root as a result of subarticular entrapment, pedicular kinking, or foramenal imingement due to posterior joint subluxation may also cause low back pain. In subarticular entrapment, hypertrophy of the superior articular facet may compress a nerve root between the facet and the dorsal aspect of the vertebral body. This occurs because nerve roots course underneath the medial border of the superior articular facet before they swing around the pedicle to emerge through the foramen.

When there is marked narrowing of the disc height, the pedicle of the upper vertebral body may kink the emerging nerve root to a significant degree if there is asymmetric collapse of the disc.

As the nerve root emerges through the foramen, it lies in close relationship to the tip of the superior facet of the vertebral body below. With disc narrowing, the posterior joints may override and the root may be, on occasion, compressed by the superior articular facet.

Congenital Conditions

Many congenital anomalies of the spinal column not involving neural elements are asymptomatic and are discovered incidentally. For example, 2% of the population have spina bifida occulta, and 6% have sacralization of a transverse process forming a pseudoarthrosis with the sacrum or the ilium without any symptoms. Most of these defects are of little or no clinical significance and require no treatment or restriction of activity. Other anomalies, initially asymptomatic, may predispose to spinal injury from relatively trivial injuries.

Scoliosis

Two types of scoliosis exist: a) nonstructural or functional scoliosis and b) structural scoliosis. A nonstructural scoliosis is a curvature that may be reversed when the individual sits or lies down. Such deformity may be due to inequality of leg length, poor posture, or protective muscle spasm in painful lesions such as sciatica.

A structural scoliosis, by contrast, is an irreversible curvature of the spine with rotation of the vertebral bodies in the area of the major curve. The most important type of structural scoliosis is idiopathic scoliosis, which accounts for about 85% of all scoliosis and is present in some degree in approximately 0.5% of the population. It is generally not a cause of back pain and progression of the curvature is unlikely.

Causes of secondary structural scoliosis include weakness of the trunk muscles from polio, hemivertebra, destructive lesions of the vertebrae, soft-tissue contractures of the chest wall, and metabolic bone disease.

In the prepubertal patient with scoliosis, the spine is x-rayed yearly for precise measurements until longitudinal growth of the spine has ceased, which is indicated by complete ossification of the iliac apophysis. During the period of observation, sleeping on a firm mattress is advised and there are no restrictions on activity. The use of therapeutic exercises is controversial.

If the curve is greater than 20° or is seen in a youngster under 10 years of age, referral to an orthopedic surgeon is indicated. Surgery for low back pain due to scoliosis is very rarely helpful, except in very few persons with lumbar scoliosis.

Leg-length discrepancy

There is no general agreement as to the significance of a leg-length discrepancy in producing symptoms of low back pain. Clinical measurements of leg length are notoriously unreliable. The standard technique of measuring the leg length from the symphysis pubis to the medial malleolus in the supine position is very dependent on the position of the pelvis. Radiological techniques are too cumbersome for routine use. A practical technique has been described on page 83.

Statistical studies suggest that differences of ½ inch or less are well within the variation between the observers and are not reliable unless based on the average of four independent measurements. Investigators have tried to make the case that differences of ¼ inch (6 mm) to a ½ inch (12.5 mm) are clinically significant and are associated with a higher prevalence of low back or leg symptoms. Other studies claim that the incidence of a short leg of ½ inch or more in the general population ranges between 4% and 8%, and is asymptomatic. When a leg-length discrepancy of greater than ½ inch is associated with chronic or recurrent low back pain, we recommend a trial with a shoe lift since it can do no harm and may be quite beneficial in some cases.

Spondylolisthesis

Spondylolisthesis is the forward displacement of one or more of the lumbar vertebrae. Spondylolisthesis may be asymptomatic or may cause backache of a mechanical type, sciatica caused by nerve-root compression from disc prolapse, or impingement by the mobile bone. Persons with spondylolisthesis frequently state that stooping relieves back pain. Five anatomical and clinical types are recognized.

Symptoms of *congenital spondylolisthesis* appear between the ages of 9 and 20. Patients should be referred to an orthopedic surgeon when there is slippage of more than one-half the diameter of the vertebral body or when there are persistent symptoms. Lumbosacral fusion appears to be a successful operation.

Spondylolytic spondylolisthesis is the most common form occurring in 5% of the population and is generally asymptomatic throughout life. The essential radiological feature is a defect or break in the pars interarticularis. It is frequently recognized incidentally on x-ray. As with most causes of back pain, conservative treatment, including lumbar support, bed rest, and modification of posture, are mandatory before surgical treatment is considered.

Traumatic spondylolisthesis implies a fracture of the base of the posterior elements running across the pars interarticularis into the pedicle with or without forward slippage. These patients are treated with a month of bed rest followed by a plaster jacket for another 3 months until healing has occurred. When union fails, surgery is indicated.

Degenerative spondylolisthesis is almost never seen in patients under 40 years old. It involves slippage between the fourth and fifth lumbar vertebrae. The high incidence of symptoms and signs is due to direct irritation and compression of the nerve roots. Individuals may have acute or chronic low back pain related to position and posture, sciatic pain with sensory and motor disturbances due to nerve root irritation and compression, or symptoms of a cauda equina syndrome. Most cases are mild and can be controlled with conservative measures. When symptoms are severe, decompression of the involved area and lumbar nerve roots may be performed.

Spinal Stenosis (Cauda Equina Compression Syndrome, Pseudoclaudication)

Spinal stenosis is an unusual but surgically treatable cause of low back and leg pain that occurs in middle-aged and elderly individuals. The possibility of spinal stenosis should always be kept in mind in the differential diagnosis of patients with claudicatory pain and intractable sciatica or back pain. Patients with spinal stenosis have been diagnosed as hysterical and malingerers, and occasionally have been operated on for arterial insufficiency.

The condition should be considered in persons with pain and/or weakness that is provoked by walking and hyperextension of the back, and is relieved by rest or flexion of the back. The pain is described as a unilateral or bilateral nagging ache, like a toothache in the calves and thighs; or tingling or burning of the feet. One third of the patients have weakness and sometimes paralysis preceded by sensory symptoms and increasing pain. Bowel and bladder sphincter disturbances and impotence occur with significant compression.

The syndrome is associated with a number of conditions that can compromise the diameter of the spinal canal:

1. Intradural or epidural tumor
2. Paget's disease
3. Intervertebral disc herniation
4. Congenital or developmental abnormalities
5. Postlumbar fusion
6. Spondylolisthesis

Physical findings are helpful if present, but their absence cannot be taken as evidence against the diagnosis. Signs of acute disc herniation are frequently absent since the neural compression is intermittent. For example, an ankle reflex present at rest may disappear after minimal exercise. The same thing applies to sensory and motor function. Many elderly patients have diminished ankle jerks and weak distal pulses, confusing the picture, with the suggestion of arterial insufficiency. In essence, the diagnosis is made on the basis of a suggestive story and myelographic findings. Plain radiographs are nondiagnostic and only suggest the diagnosis. Magnetic resonance imaging, computed tomography, or myelography are the most useful diagnostic tests if surgery is contemplated. The results of back surgery, usually a generous laminectomy and decompression of nerve roots, show that two-thirds to three-fourths of operated persons will have relief of incapacitating pain, one-half will have some residual back pain postoperatively, and only 15% will have persistent pain with longer follow-up. In general, though symptom relief may not be complete, it is significant enough to improve functional capacity.

Management of Mechanical Back Pain

The management of low back pain includes modalities from manipulation to surgery. Reasonably well-controlled studies, albeit with a small number of subjects, all demonstrate that few of the treatments presently available are superior to time and bed rest. Regardless of the treatment, be it manipulation, traction, or bed rest, three-quarters of persons may be expected to get well within 3 weeks and 90% within 2 months. Deyo has critically reviewed clinical trials of low back pain treatment and only 8 of 59 studies fulfilled requirements for scientific validity.

The key to treatment of low back pain is bed rest, which markedly reduces intradiscal pressure. Antiinflammatory agents, analgesics, and muscle relaxants contribute marginally to bed rest. Wiesel et al. compared Army recruits treated either by strict bed rest or ambulation. The bed rest group was functional in 6.6 days versus 11.8 days for the ambulatory group, regardless of the severity of pain. The addition of aspirin, phenylbutazone, acetaminophen with codeine, or oxycodone with aspirin did not alter the functional outcome, but patients reported less pain. It has also been shown that short-term bed rest is effective. Deyo compared the effects of 2 versus 7 days of bed rest. The shorter treatment resulted in 45% less time lost from work and there were no differences in patient perception of treatment effect or their functional capacity both 3 weeks and 3 months later.

Pain control

The contribution of antiinflammatory agents and analgesic medication in the treatment of acute low back pain is probably marginal. In the study cited above, analgesic medication combined with bed rest further decreased the amount of pain, particularly when used in the first 3 days of the onset. However, analgesic medication did not allow a more prompt return to work. There are no data to suggest that a particular analgesic is superior to others or that the ritual of prescribing a muscle relaxant is really necessary. Aspirin or the equivalent with or without codeine for 3 to 5 days is sufficient analgesia.

Methocarbarmol (Robaxin®), carisoprodol (Soma®), and similar drugs promoted as muscle relaxants do not have a specific effect on neuromuscular junctions, and whatever effects they have on muscle tone are probably due to depressant effects on the central nervous system. Their effectiveness in relieving back pain is no greater than that of ordinary sedatives.

Oral benzodiazepines, particularly diazepam (Valium®), have been widely recommended for their muscle-relaxing properties. In controlled clinical trials of benzodiazepines in musculoskeletal disorders, diazepam is superior to other muscle relaxants (chlormezanone, carisoprodol, methocarbarmol), but diazepam in relatively low doses is not consistently different from placebo or aspirin. It is likely that favorable results with this drug are due to the natural history of the condition and the combined effect of rest and nonspecific central effects.

Putting a person with acute back pain to bed with firm support (i.e., a bed board) and with hips flexed relieves pain and muscle spasm. Unfortunately, this prescription may be difficult to follow because of work, family, or other pressures. Hospitalization or home care may be necessary if bed rest cannot be accomplished.

Which patients need to be put to bed? Certainly, a patient with evidence of nerve-root compression. Other candidates include the person with acute muscle spasm and compensatory scoliosis, the person who has not responded to ambulatory treatment, and the person who has not responded to conservative therapy and is considering surgery.

If the patient is put to bed, isometric exercises of the abdominal muscles and hamstring stretching should be advised.

Patient education for prevention

An important task in managing chronic or recurrent back pain of any cause is to provide instructions on how to minimize stress on the spine (Table 4–5). Erect, the body's weight is transmitted to the intervertebral discs and particularly on the posterior edges of the discs. Minimizing lordosis reduces these forces, and the essential lesson for individuals with low back pain is to sit, stand, walk, and lie in positions that minimize the lordosis of the back. Factors that contribute to extension of the spine, such as weak abdominal muscles, tight hamstrings, obesity, and high heels should be corrected.

Studies suggest that strong muscles protect the back from painful episodes. Individuals with low back pain have weaker abdominal muscles than those with no back pain. In all age groups, inactivity of longer than 1 month results in diminished abdominal and extensor strength. A recent prospective study of firefighters suggests that fitness decreases one's susceptibility to back injuries.

In lifting or carrying heavy objects, increased intraabdominal and intrathoracic pressure resulting from contraction of muscles normally relieves some of the load imposed on the spine. Lifting with the knees flexed, forward bending with weight in the hands, sit-ups, and active back hyperextension all increase the intradiscal pressure to nearly 200% of that observed while standing. Walking, twisting, and straining cause only modest increases, and isometric contraction of the abdominal muscles causes no greater increase than laughing. Straight stand-

TABLE 4–5. PATIENT EDUCATION — CARING FOR YOUR BACK

Always remember to sit, stand, and lie in positions that flatten the hollow in your low back.

The back muscles and stomach muscles oppose each other. If the stomach muscles are weak, the back muscles will increase the hollow in the low back and put pressure on the backbones (vertebrae) and the discs. Pelvic tilt exercises draw the back of the pelvis down and the front of the pelvis up, which tends to reduce the hollow in the back. Prolonged standing should be avoided. With prolonged standing, one unconsciously tries to avoid fatigue and relaxes the muscles that support the low back and, thereby, shifts the weight backwards and increases the pressure on the back of the lower lumbar vertebrae. In standing, the body weight should be supported primarily on the heels, and the chest should be shifted slightly forward so a crease is formed across the upper abdomen. Both knees should be flexed slightly. Shortening of the abdominal muscles pulls the chest forward and relieves the pressure on the lower spine.

Standing and walking should be done with the toes pointed straightforward. Standing with the toes pointed forward increased the base of support from front to back.

High heels cause the body to tilt forward, unless the trunk is bent backward.

Overweight and pregnant individuals carry an extra load in front and the spine is thrown back. These conditions make these guidelines difficult, but if you are conscious of your posture and work on making your stomach muscles stronger, you can do much to reduce pain.

General Exercise

When you have back trouble or are prone to having back trouble, be sensible about how you treat it. Swimming, especially back stroking, and walking are useful ways to keep fit without stressing the back.

Sitting

Sitting with the hollow in the low back flattened is an effective way to ease low back pain. The key to comfortable sitting lies in the elevation of the knees above the hips. This stretches the spine and reduces pressure on any nerve roots. This is particularly important in setting the position of the driver's seat.

Lying Down

Lying on the stomach usually makes back pain worse, whereas, lying on the back on a firm mattress with the hips and knees each bent to 90° eases pressure and pain. The most comfortable sleeping position for most people is on the back with the knees propped up or on-the-side with the knees drawn up. A firm mattress or a mattress with a bed board underneath presses the buttock and the back of the pelvis forward, thus diminishing the hollow in the low back.

Lifting and Carrying

Lifting should be done with the legs rather than the back. Don't bend over with the legs straight to pick up heavy objects, but take the weight with your legs bent and hold the object close to your body (to reduce the leverage of the weight).

Approach the object straight on. Embrace the object. Tighten your stomach muscles as you stand up with the object.

ing is better than unsupported sitting, and activities such as walking and twisting are less stressful than straining, coughing, and jumping.

Individuals should avoid prolonged standing. With prolonged standing, one unconsciously relaxes the muscles that support the back and, thereby, shifts the weight to the posterior edges of the vertebrae. In standing, the weight should be taken on the heels, with the knees flexed and the abdominal muscles contracted

TABLE 4–6. DISTINGUISHING FEATURES OF MECHANICAL VERSUS INFLAMMATORY BACK PAIN

Clinical Features	Mechanical	Inflammatory
Discomfort	Episodic	Persistent
Onset	Acute	Insidious
Age (years)	15 to 90	40
Morning stiffness	+	+++
Involvement of other systems	Absent	Eyes, joints, skin, lungs
Effect of exercise	Worse	Better
Effect of rest	Better	Worse
Radiation of pain	Anatomic (S1, L5)	Diffuse (thoracic, buttock)
Sensory symptoms	Present	Absent
Motor symptoms	Present	Absent
Decreased range of movement	Asymmetrical	Symmetrical
Tenderness	Local	Diffuse

to splint the lower spine; putting one foot on the bar rail or on a short stool accomplishes the same. High heels tilt the body forward, which is compensated by increased lordosis and should be avoided.

Sitting should be done with good lumbar support with the knees and hips flexed. In the absence of support, slumping, which may be considered uncouth in certain circles, or wrapping one's legs around the legs of the chair, straightens the spine.

Forward bending, for prolonged periods should be avoided. Patients should be shown how to lift objects with their legs rather than with flexing the back and to "hug" the object. The difference in load on the disc between lifting 20 kg close to the body compared with lifting the same weight at arm's length is about 150 kg in individuals of slim build.

The advice to take care of one's back may be taken to mean that avoidance of certain activities will prevent damage and the person may turn himself or herself into an invalid. If this inactivity continues for more than a couple of months, the pattern is difficult to break. An explicit program of progressive activity must be outlined, and a referral to physical therapy is the best way to accomplish this.

Therapeutic exercises (Table 4–7)

Many exercises actually increase loading forces on the spine and raise intradiscal pressures to magnitudes as high as those measured in standing and leaning forward with weights in the hands. If patients do not point out exercises that make them worse, they may simply not comply.

Isometric exercises improve the strength of the abdominal muscles and give better results than flexion and extension exercises.

Intermittent traction, exercises for all ranges of motion and muscle groups, manipulation by the Maitland technique, corsets, and combinations of the above appear to have no beneficial effects that are detectable at 4 or 16 months, although active physiotherapy appears to have some small value in patients with sciatica in the short term.

Written, illustrated material is useful for teaching persons about specific

TABLE 4–7. PATIENT EDUCATION — LOW BACK EXERCISES

Painful Stage

1. Pelvic tilt: With knees bent, tilt pelvis up by tightening abdominal muscles and squeezing buttock muscles together, flattening small of back down against floor. Hold position for 10 seconds. Repeat ______ times. Then relax.
2. Same starting position as #1. Pull one leg gently to chest helping with hands. Return leg to bent-knee position. Relax and repeat with opposite leg. Repeat ______ times.
3. Sitting in chair with legs apart and feet on floor. Bend forward and dangle arms between legs gently, attempting to touch floor. Return to sitting position. Return ______ times.
4. Getting out of bed. Move close to edge of bed. Turn on your side and bend your hips and knees. Let your lower legs swing over the side of the bed and push with the arm that is closest to the bed. This will bring you to a sitting position with feet on the floor.
5. Standing from bed or chair. Make sure feet are flat on the floor. Lean forward but do not bend over. Push with arms and straighten knees to come to standing. Tighten buttocks to bring you erect.

After Painful Stage

1. Lie on back, bend hips and knees until feet are flat on bed or floor; grab both knees with hands and bring knees to chest. At the same time, curl head down toward knees. Hold for count of 3. Return to starting position. Repeat ______ times.
2. Same starting position as #1 above. Place hands on thighs and try to sit up keeping knees bent and feet flat on bed. If unable to sit up, use arms to assist sitting up, making sure arms do as little work as possible. Your stomach muscles should shake. Never do these exercises by anchoring your feet or having someone hold your feet, as this maneuver pulls the front of the pelvis down, increasing the hollow in the back.

exercises, but most persons need to be taken through the drills. Very obese or flabby individuals will have difficulty doing a proper pelvic tilt because their muscle tone is so poor that any proprioceptive notion of their abdominal muscles contracting has faded. Life-long habits of poor posture or body mechanics that stress the spine cannot be changed by a pamphlet. Special instruction supervised by a physiotherapist is needed.

Mobilization and manipulation are maneuvers applied manually to the lumbar area, consisting either of repetitive oscillatory movements (mobilization) or increasingly forceful thrusts (manipulation). There is no evidence that techniques recommended for correcting malalignment or reducing disc bulging work.

Short-term manipulation may temporarily decrease pain and improve function, but has little or no lasting benefit. There is no evidence that manipulation for more than 2 weeks results in sustained pain relief or improved function. There are reports of forceful manipulation causing new or increased neurological deficits.

A few patients respond quickly to manipulation, but there is no way of identifying such patients in advance, although painful limitation of extension may be such a feature that predicts beneficial results. Rotational manipulation in patients with uncomplicated low back pain and no contraindications tends to result in immediate relief after the first treatment, but no long-term benefit has been demonstrated. Studies show that there is no point in continuing to manipulate patients who show no early improvement.

Another variant of manipulative therapy is traction, which can be applied by autotraction, gravity reduction, or motorized devices. At least 60% of body weight must be applied before the lumbar disc changes its dimensions. Claims that disc herniations can be reduced are unproven. Two studies have shown that autotraction is superior to either corset or sham treatment in low back pain and sciatica, but that the effect is short lived. Another study showed no benefits of tratcion and bed rest compared to bed rest alone, and concluded that traction simply reinforced the need for rest.

Low back supports (braces and corsets)

If the supporting muscles of the spine are stripped away, the heaviest load that the spine can sustain in the vertical position without buckling is four or five pounds. During some strenuous physical activity, stresses far exceeding the required force to fracture a vertebra are sustained. That we do not regularly buckle or break our backs is due to the contraction of the trunk muscles, which increases intraabdominal pressure, reduces the load on the lumbar discs, and transforms the stack of bones and discs into a rigid structure. Corsets and braces reduce vertical loading forces by abdominal compression, which diminishes the load on the spine and discs by 30% to 50%.

During normal lifting, trunk muscles contract proportionally to the load being lifted. When a corset is applied, the normal activity of the muscle is diminished. Therefore, a corset begets disuse atrophy and ineffective "splinting" of the spine. Corsets and braces should be used only as temporary measures.

A brace or a corset limits spinal motion, corrects posture, reduces mechanical stress on the lumbosacral spine, and "reminds" a patient to avoid extension stress on the back. A brace and corset are alike in every respect with the exception that a brace has rigid horizontal elements. In general, a brace limits all motion to a greater degree, but a corset is lighter and better tolerated.

Corsets are constructed of reinforced fabric with flexible or rigid stays and are adjusted by side or back lacing. One type consists of a molded plastic insert that fits into an abdominal binder.

Spinal supports facilitate an earlier return to functional activities for patients with slowly subsiding acute mechanical low back pain. All patients who get a spine support should exercise the abdominal musculature to avoid weakening of the muscles. A spine support should not be worn longer than 4 hours a day.

Extradural injections

Extradural injections of local anesthetic with or without steroids are a valuable addition to the management of disc disease and are easy to administer in an outpatient setting. A few patients respond dramatically, some are partially helped, and many others get transitory relief. In chronic sciatica, steroid injections may give relief in patients with intractable pain that is resistant to other treatments.

Corticosteroids

Oral dexamethasone has also been used in the management of patients with herniated lumbar discs. Green described 100 consecutive patients with radicular pain due to myelographically proven herniated lumbar intervertebral discs who were treated with dexamethasone (64 mg on day 1, 32 mg on day 2, 24 mg on day 3, 12 mg on day 4, and 8 mg on days 5 through 7). All patients had relief of pain within 24 to 48 hours. Before treatment with dexamethasone, 15 of the patients had been treated with bed rest alone from 7 to 21 days without satisfactory relief of pain.

During the initial hours of treatment, all patients noted a marked decrease in pain, which was manifested not only in their subjective response but also in diminished pain medication requirements. Nine patients required surgery during the 15 months of follow-up. Review of work status and recurrent pain during the follow-up period indicated that the nonsurgically treated patients did better. Although uncontrolled, the results are impressive and should be confirmed in a randomized, controlled study.

Surgery

Surgery for low back pain should be considered in the patient with demonstrable segmental instability from spondylolisthesis, spinal stenosis, lumbar scoliosis, and the patient with a herniated disc who has failed conservative treatment. For most patients with low back pain from a degenerated disc, surgery is not indicated. Even in 70% of persons with a clear-cut herniated disc, conservative treatment with bed rest and analgesics is sufficient.

One retrospective and one prospective, randomized trial have compared operative to nonoperative treatment in patients with lumbar disc herniation and sciatica. Weber's study showed that at 1 and 2 years, greater function and fewer symptoms were reported by the operatively treated patients without cauda equina lesions or paresis, but 4 and 10 years later, both groups had comparable function and complaints.

The only absolute indication for lumbar disc surgery is a midline disc herniation with progressive neurologic deficits. The majority of back surgery is done for relative indications. These include failure to respond to conservative medical management, recurrent back pain, or intractable sciatica interfering with function.

The choice of a particular operation appears to be much less important than patient selection. Patients at particular risk for a poor result can be predicted by the physical findings which suggest psychological disturbances, by pending workman's compensation claims, and by the Minnesota Multiphasic Personality Inventory (MMPI) showing a profile of hysteria, hypochondriasis, and somatisization. Conversely, unequivocal clinical signs and symptoms, and computed tomography scans or myelograms that are consistent with symptoms and signs, are associated with a high probability of success. In patients with these favorable features, surgery may still be delayed for up to 12 weeks to see if improvement occurs. Further delay may compromise the outcome, particularly if there is muscular weakness or paresis.

In a patient with confirmed disc herniation, surgery that is delayed for 5 months or more gives less successful results. In properly timed surgical removal of a prolapsed disc, 7 to 8 out of 10 patients will obtain complete relief of sciatica and approximately two thirds will also be relieved of back pain. Naylor found postoperative backache occurring in 17% of his series. Hakelius followed two groups of patients, one treated conservatively and the other surgically, and showed that in the conservatively managed group, backache persisted in 31% as compared with 26% of those treated surgically.

The complications of surgery include persistent or recurrent back pain, infection of the intervertebral disc space (in less than 1% of operations), vascular injuries during the operation, and development of meningeal pseudocysts.

Discectomy may be done by a variety of approaches, but the goal is to decompress the involved nerve root(s), while maintaining spinal stability. Five to 15 percent of patients subsequently require further surgery for a variety of reasons, most commonly a recurrent disc herniation. The disc removal can also be performed by using cutting and suctioning instruments placed through a percutaneous approach. Early uncontrolled clinical trials indicate that this technique can relieve sciatica in 60% to 80% of patients. This technique is largely confined ot the L4–L5 disc because of anatomical impediments to needle placement at other levels. Microscopic discectomy uses smaller incisions to accomplish the same goals. Proponents of this technique cite less postoperative pain, while detractors cite a higher rate of recurrent symptoms from missed disc fragments.

Chemonucleolysis

Chymopapain is reported to relieve sciatica in 58% to 90% of treated patients. Two studies show that about 80% of patients treated with chymopapain and 50% of controls have relief 6 weeks after injection. The enthusiasm for chymopapain has waned because of complications such as transverse myelitis (1/1000 injections), allergic reactions (0.5%), and persisting low back pain (20%). Comparisons of chymopapain to surgical removal of discs indicate a more predictable early relief of sciatica with surgery, although the results 10 years after the intervention appear comparable.

INFLAMMATORY BACK PAIN

Soft-Tissue Syndromes

When a deep structure of the back is irritated by trauma, disease, or inflammation, the resulting pain may be felt locally, referred distally, or a combination of both. For instance, if hypertonic saline is injected in the supraspinous ligament between T12 and L1, pain is felt in the low back, both buttocks, and as low as the greater trochanter. A similar injection between L5 and S1 gives rise to buttock pain and pain down the posterior leg, which rarely goes below the knee, but occasionally may extend to the ankle, mimicking sciatica. Such pain may also be associated with tender points over the sacroiliac joint or the upper quadrant of the buttock. Thus, local tenderness does not necessarily mean that the spot is the culprit, even if temporary relief is afforded by local injection of an anesthetic agent; tenderness as well as pain can be referred.

Sprains or strains of muscle cause local tenderness and pain, usually lasting no more than 3 weeks if the person does not aggravate the original injury by injudicious activities. In the young person, muscle and ligamentous injury occurs as an isolated event, whereas a similar injury in an older person may also injure a joint.

Partial tears of muscle attachments cause local tenderness and pain. With time, the lesions heal. Such measures as local injections of anesthetic with or without corticosteroids may afford temporary relief, but probably do not speed the healing process. Generally, symptoms may persist for up to 3 weeks, and if pain persists beyond this, the patient should be reassessed.

Tendinitis is thought to be due to localized tendon degeneration that invokes an inflammatory response. Tendinous attachments to the sacrum or iliac crest and supraspinous ligaments may be particularly vulnerable. Tendinitis causes diffuse vague backache that is aggravated with repetitive motions of the back. The diagnosis is made when point tenderness is elicited at the site of a tendinous insertion and reproduces the person's symptoms. Local injections of anesthetic and/or corticosteroids may give rapid pain relief.

Sprains and instability of the sacroiliac joints may present as back pain. A sprain of the sacroiliac joint, other than in latter months of pregnancy and violent trauma, is rare. Less than 2% of acute back pain is due to problems of the sacroiliac joint. The sacroiliac joint, held by powerful ligaments, is extremely sturdy. Under 45 years of age, minimal movement may occur with normal activity, but major force must be applied to move the joints beyond their anatomical limits. In the age group most vulnerable to backache, the over 45-year-old group, a third of the population have ossified the anterior capsule, which virtually excludes the sacroiliac joints as the cause of backache.

Pathology of the sacroiliac joint is suspected when the symptoms are reproduced by maneuvers that stress the joint:

1. Compression of the iliac crest in the lateral decubitus position moves the sacroiliac joint, as the pelvis is a closed ring.
2. Resisted abduction of the hip on the side of the pain requires that the gluteus medius contract, which pulls the ilium away from the sacrum.
3. Hyperextending the hip on the symptomatic side with the other hip flexed, and thus stabilized, will produce pain only with sacroiliac disease, hip pathology, or fourth nerve-root irritation.

Myofascial Syndromes

Myalgia, fibromyalgia, fibrositis, fibromyositis, myofibrositis, fasciitis, myofascitis, and muscular rheumatism describe syndromes of musculoskeletal pain with no characteristic laboratory or histological abnormalities. No "typical" history exists. The onset may be associated with acute muscular strain, a febrile illness, or chronic infection, or it may develop insidiously. Pain is described as knifelike, stabbing or shooting, dull or aching. Muscle stiffness after rest, fatigue (frequently on awakening), and/or sleep disturbance suggest depression, but the patient may not have any functional impairment.

Of the theories put forth to explain the syndrome, there is but little circumstantial evidence that the underlying lesion is inflamed connective tissue, local hypoxia of the muscle, sustained muscular contraction, referred pain from a distant source, an allergic or autoimmune phenomena, or a psychophysiological condition.

A cardinal feature of muscle pain syndromes is palpable hardening of the involved muscles, which are usually painful. In back pain, these might be nodules of the gluteus maximus and medius, the quadratus lumborum, iliocostal, longissimus, and multifidus. These painful nodules or trigger points may be associated with cutaneous hyperalgesia.

Treatment of various soft-tissue lesions is empirical and includes trigger point injection, massage, etc. Myofascial syndromes of the back are treated empirically with injections of local anesthetic or spraying ethyl chloride on the involved area. The response is unpredictable and normal saline injections are reported to be effective as well. Aerobic conditioning helps many patients. Passive stretching of the involved area, moist heat, cold, diathermy, ultrasound, and other local approaches have been promoted. Antiinflammatory agents and analgesics are not generally helpful. Antidepressants used to treat the sleep disturbance seen in many patients is helpful at doses that are frequently not adequate to treat depression. Amitryptyline from 12.5 mg to 50 mg is the usual dosage range.

Sacroiliitis

The possibility of an inflammatory lesion of the sacroiliac joint in back pain of obscure pathology needs to be kept in mind in individuals with:

1. A history of insidious onset of back stiffness or backache before age 30
2. Back stiffness for more than 30 minutes on awakening
3. Symptoms that are improved with activity
4. Psoriasis, uveitis or iritis, urethritis, or inflammatory bowel disease

Some distinguishing features of inflammatory back disease from mechanical causes are given in Table 4–6.

Sacroiliitis is seen in ankylosing spondylitis, spondylitis associated with psoriatic arthritis, Reiter's syndrome, ileal bypass surgery, and inflammatory bowel disease with or without peripheral joint involvement. Ninety percent or more of individuals with ankylosing spondylitis and Reiter's syndrome are HLA B27 positive (in contrast, approximately 8% of a normal Caucasian population are HLA B27 positive).

The spondylitis associated with inflammatory bowel disease and psoriasis appears to progress independently of the bowel or skin disease, whereas the activity of the peripheral arthropathy in these conditions tends to correlate with the activity of the primary disease.

The triad of Reiter's syndrome is nonbacterial urethritis, arthritis, and conjunctivitis. A number of patients show radiographic evidence of sacroiliitis but only a small percentage have clinically significant spondylitis.

The sacroiliac joint is lined by synovium only in the lower two-thirds; the upper third is held together by interosseous ligaments. Aside from suspecting sacroiliitis on clinical grounds, a posteroanterior x-ray view of the pelvis will show erosive changes, pseudowidening from erosion, and subchondral sclerosis on the iliac *and* sacral sides of the joint.

Changes by technetium scans and computed tomography precede those of plain x-rays but are not generally available. In cases where there is strong suspicion of spondylitis and the x-rays appear normal, radiological examination should be repeated. The natural history of spondylitic syndromes may take months to years before the diagnosis is obvious by x-ray.

Myelitis

The spinal cord may be the target of infection and noninfective inflammatory processes, affecting primarily the neurons, meninges, myelin, or combinations thereof. Meningomyelitis due to syphilis, tuberculosis, or suppurative infections is rare but treatable. Meningomyelitis generally causes symptoms of burning and stinging or back pain with constitutional symptoms. Numbness occurs in a distribution of one or more sensory nerve roots and becomes bilateral, persistent, and unchanged by movement or straining. Symptoms of root involvement precede signs of cord compression by months or years. Sooner or later, if the process is unchecked, progressive spastic ataxia with sphincteric involvement results.

Inflammation of myelitis after infections and vaccinations, myelitis in multiple sclerosis, and degenerative myelitis usually presents with weakness, numbness, or paralysis of the lower extremity, and not as back pain, usually.

The diagnosis of these conditions is made by examination of the cerebrospinal fluid and appropriate cultures. Treatment consists of appropriate antibiotic therapy and corticosteroids. Myelitis due to polio, *herpes zoster*, rabies, and monkey B virus are incurable and management is supportive. Back pain is usually a minor component of these infections, the diagnosis of which becomes clear with observation.

Infections

Infections of the elements of the spine are rare but potentially treatable. Delay in recognition can lead to sepsis or irreversible neurological deficits. Backache is the most common presentation of vertebral osteomyelitis, intervertebral disc space infection, and spinal epidural abscess. Early in the course, the pain may be indistinguishable from common mechanical causes of back pain. With progression of the disease, however, the pain becomes severe, constant, and aggravated by the least amount of spinal movements (landing on one's heels, for example). The course from onset of back pain to the point of such pain, fever, constitutional symptoms, and neurological deficits may be as short as 1 to 3 days in an epidural abscess; or weeks to months in the case of osteomyelitis of the spine with slow-growing organisms, such as tuberculosis or fungal infections. With mycotic or tuberculous infections, the first symptom may be a major neurological deficit. The causes of spine infections have changed since the introduction of antimicrobials, but the predominant organism is still staphylococcus.

Fever is almost always present if there is an abscess. Any person with back pain, fever, and local spine tenderness should be assumed to have either spinal epidural abscess, infection of the vertebral body or disc space, an intraspinal tumor, a vascular accident of the spinal cord, or an acute transverse myelopathy; and needs to be hospitalized for diagnosis and treatment.

Physical findings depend on the stage and the anatomical location of the infection. Severe paravertebral muscle spasm, local spine tenderness over spinous processes, and focal neurological deficits are seen. Occasionally, a tender mass can be palpated posteriorly or a psoas abscess can be detected. The white blood cell count can be normal, but the sedimentation rate is usually elevated. Bone scanning is more sensitive to osseous destruction than plain radiographs. Radiological features begin weeks after the onset of infection with localized osteoporosis of the vertebral end plates followed by involvement of the adjacent vertebrae and narrowing of the disc spaces; and much later, with erosion and reactive sclerosis, and periosteal bone formation of contiguous vertebral bodies.

Infections of the sacroiliac joint are rare. Tuberculosis was the most common infective agent in the past, but pyogenic bacteria is now the most common etiological agent. The patient with sacroiliac infection is ill, febrile, and complains of back pain. Local tenderness may not be present but maneuvers that move the joint will produce pain.

Management of Inflammatory Back Pain

Infections of the spine are treated by specific antibiotic therapy and thus require hospitalization. For sacroiliitis, antiinflammatory agents such as indomethacin and phenylbutazone are the most useful. In ankylosing spondylitis, referral to a rheumatologist for supervised physiotherapy is indicated to ensure that when ankylosis occurs, the spine will be in the best functional position. Regular monitoring of the spine movements is necessary. It is not known whether spondylitis in any of the known syndromes is arrested by the use of antiinflammatory agents.

BACK PAIN FROM LESIONS OF BONE

Tumor

Tumors of bone may present with pain in the absence of objective neurological deficits. The most common lesions of the spinal canal are neurofibroma and ependymoma, and of the spine itself are metastatic carcinoma (lung, breast, prostate, kidney, and thyroid) and multiple myeloma.

Benign tumors occur most frequently in individuals under 30 and are likely to be asymptomatic. Hemangiomas, aneurysmal bone cysts, osteoid osteomas, eosinophilic granuloma, giant cell tumor, osteochondroma, and chondromas are the principal tumors encountered in descending order of frequency. These tumors generally follow a benign course, but may weaken the bone and produce symptoms of backache accompanied by painful scoliosis. Since idiopathic scoliosis is rarely accompanied by severe pain or symptoms until the person attains adulthood, the possibility of a benign tumor must be considered in a young person with painful scoliosis.

Hemangiomas of the vertebral body can be demonstrated radiographically as a vertebra with a honeycombed or corduroy appearance in 4% of the population. Hemangioma occurs no more frequently in a backache population and implies that other causes of back pain must be excluded first. Osteoid osteomas present with progressive back pain and may be severe enough to disturb sleep. Eighty percent of the patients are between ages 5 and 25. The typical lesion on x-ray is that of a central radiolucent area with a halo of dense sclerosis. Pain from osteomas respond to nonsteroidal antiinflammatory agents.

When back pain occurs for the first time in an individual under age 30 (primary tumor) or over 50 (metastatic disease), especially without a clear history of a precipitating activity or pain relieved by rest, the possibility of a tumor should be entertained. Table 4–8 compares clinical features of tumor versus mechanical back pain, but overlap occurs. Roentgenographic examinations of the area are the least sensitive, as more than 50% of the bony mass must be destroyed before changes are apparent. Bone scanning is the most sensitive and efficient way to define a tumor lesion. For myeloma, however, the plain x-ray is more sensitive than bone scan. For intraspinal tumors, myelography, computed tomography (CT), and magnetic resonance imaging (MRI) allow visualization of the area. The disadvantage of magnetic resonance imaging is cost.

Metabolic Bone Disease

Disorders of bone, osteoporosis, osteomalacia, hyperparathyroidism, Paget's disease, osteopetrosis, and alkaptonuria may present as back pain. Nothing in the history or physical examination particularly distinguishes bone pain from other causes of back pain. The diagnosis is suggested by the x-ray of the lumbosacral spine, which shows osteopenia, the differential diagnosis of which includes idiopathic osteoporosis, osteomalacia, hyperparathyroidism, hyperthyroidism, and diffuse osteolytic metastases. Paget's disease and the exceedingly rare syndromes, osteopetrosis and akaptonuria, each have their own characteristic radiological features. Of these, osteoporosis is by far the most common. The physiology of bone pain in osteoporosis without a fracture is obscure, but it may be due to increased pressure within the vertebrae itself from increased vascularity.

TABLE 4–8. TUMOR VERSUS MECHANIC CAUSE OF BACK PAIN

Tumor	Mechanic
Onset at age < 30 or > 50	Age of onset between 30 and 50
Constitutional symptoms (fever, weight loss)	No constitutional symptoms
Sudden onset of pain without history of precipitants	History of precipitants
Progressive pain or radiculopathy refractory to treatment	Clinical improvement with conservative therapy
Pain bilateral	
Pain pattern changed	
Pain with bed rest and hips flexed	Pain relieved by rest, aggravated by activity
Pseudoclaudication	
Known primary cancer	
Midline abnormalities on exam (pain, Faun's beard, hemangioma, palpable mass)	
Elevated sedimentation rate	Normal sedimentation rate
Elevated alkaline phosphatase	Normal alkaline phosphatase

Management of Back Pain from Bone Sources (see Chapter 12)

The treatment of primary and secondary bone tumors requires consultation and usually hospitalization. Painful metastatic tumor of the spine may be treated symptomatically (indomethacin seems to be particularly useful for this indication) or with radiation therapy. If signs of myelopathy are present, urgent operative decompression is necessary.

The major goal in managing osteoporosis is its prevention, because when symptomatic osteoporosis occurs or osteopenia is present on x-ray, nearly 30% to 50% of the bone mass has been lost. Preventive therapy might be directed at populations at highest risk for osteoporosis: postmenopausal, white, sedentary, thin-boned, non-milk-drinking women who avoid sunlight or those on long courses of corticosteroids. Important nonmedical strategies include ensuring maximal development of skeletal mass during growth periods, encouraging exercise, and graded exposure to sunlight. Conjugated estrogens given at the time of normal or surgical menopause in a dose of 0.625 mg is associated with a fivefold reduction in the incidence of vertebral compression fractures and stabilization of bone mass. The increased risk of endometrial carcinoma associated with estrogen use needs to be considered. Calcium in a dose of 1 g daily with vitamin D, 50,000 IU twice weekly, are claimed to decrease bone lost in patients on long-term corticosteroids or patients who have poor dietary patterns. Sodium fluoride is still investigational in the long-term treatment of osteoporosis. Calcium intake and absorption tend to decline with age, and women over 40 should receive at least 750 mg of calcium in their diet per day (one glass of skim milk, one tablespoon of Titratac, and one TUMS ($CaCo_3$) each contain 250 mg of calcium).

In patients who have sustained vertebral crush fractures, bed rest and analgesics are needed during the acute phase (7 to 10 days), but the patient should be gotten up as soon as it is feasible, since immobilization is a potent leacher of bone mass.

REFERRED BACK PAIN

Back pain may be referred from the kidneys, female reproductive organs, and retroperitoneal structures (pancreas, abdominal aorta, etc.), but backache is seldom the only symptom of these disorders. Peptic ulceration or tumor of the stomach and duodenal ulcer typically induce pain in the epigastrium. If posterior wall involvement or retroperitoneal extension exists, pain may be felt in the back. If the back pain is due to peptic ulceration, it occurs hours after a meal and is relieved by food and antacids.

Diseases of the pancreas (peptic ulceration with extension to the pancreas, cholecystitis with pancreatitis, tumor) can cause pain in the back, being more to the right of the spine if the head of the pancreas is involved, and to the left if the body and tail are implicated.

Conditions in the retroperitoneum, e.g., lymphomas and sarcomas, evoke back pain, sometimes radiating to the lower abdomen, groin, and anterior thigh. A tumor in the iliopsoas region produce unilateral lumbar ache with radiation toward the groin and labia or testicles, with occasional evidence of involvement of the upper lumbar spinal roots.

Inflammatory diseases of the colon (colitis, diverticulitis) or tumor of the colon produce pain between the umbilicus and pubis, in the midlumbar region, or in both. A lesion of the transverse colon or first part of the descending colon may be central or left-sided, referring to second to third lumbar vertebrae. If the sigmoid colon is involved, pain refers to the upper sacral region and anteriorly to the suprapubic region or left lower quadrant of the abdomen.

The single most important historical feature that distinguishes pathology in the spine due to referred pain from abdominal organs is the fact that the pain is *not* aggravated by activity, nor is it relieved by rest.

Gynecologic disorders may manifest themselves as back pain. Low back pain is manifested in many women with dysmennorrhea as heaviness, fullness, or vague pelvic ache. During pregnancy, softening of ligaments combined with weakened, stretched abdominal muscles and stress on the spine from increased lordosis contribute to the common occurrence of low back pain as well as sciatica. For most expectant mothers, the discomfort is of minimal concern compared with the excitement of the forthcoming event. In others, great expectations are not enough and pain can be severe, requiring bed rest. Medications should be avoided; sciatica of pregnancy can be relieved temporarily by assuming an "all-fours" position on the hands and knees.

The most important source of chronic back pain from the pelvis is the uterosacral ligaments. Endometriosis or carcinoma of the uterus (body or cervix) may invade these structures, while malposition of the uterus may pull on them. The pain is localized centrally in the sacrum below the lumbosacral joint, but may be more on one side. In endometriosis, the pain begins during the premenstrual phase and often continues until it merges with menstrual pain. Malposition of the uterus (retroversion and prolapse) lead to sacral pain, especially after the patient has been standing for several hours. Fibroids are common but are an uncommon cause of low back pain.

Prostatitis, evidenced by a discharge, burning, and frequency of urination may be attended by a nagging sacral ache. The ache may be one sided, with radiation into one leg if the seminal vesicle is involved on that side.

An abdominal aortic aneurysm, which impinges or erodes the spine, produces boring lumbar pain unrelated to activity. Inadequate flow through the superior gluteal artery may give rise to buttock pain, which is precipitated by walking, is relieved in seconds by stopping, and is not aggravated by activities that put stress on the spine, such as bending. In an acute dissection of the abdominal aorta, the patient almost always describes acute severe pain that is maximal and constant, and is not related to movement of the spine. The only exception may be patients with Marfan's syndrome or similar disorders of connective tissue who can have dissection with mild-to-moderate pain.

PSYCHOGENIC BACK PAIN

Some patients with chronic pain become preoccupied with the symptoms to the exclusion of everything else, view themselves as a suffering invalid, and develop noncoping, dependent lifestyles. Psychological factors also aggravate existing pain. For instance, low back pain can be due largely to muscle spasm provoked by emotional problems, and its presence may add to the individual's anxiety increasing muscle tension, thus further intensifying the pain. This vicious cycle may develop a life of its own, and thus pain can be perpetuated long after the original noxious stimuli has passed.

Pain viewed from the model of operant conditioning postulates that behavior is influenced by reinforcing consequences. Thus, if behavior is followed by positive reinforcement, the behavior will be increased and persist. If the behavior is followed by negative reinforcement, the behavior will diminish irrespective of the underlying disease process. In persons with chronic disease, recognition of this phenomena may be helpful in preventing prolonged disability. The degree to which organic and psychological aspects operate in a given patient may vary from time to time, although as time increases, psychological aspects dominate.

Therapeutic objectives should emphasize activity rather than feelings of pain. Instead of asking, "How are you?" or "How do you feel?", ask about activity, "What did you do yesterday?" or "How much have you been able to do?" or "How far can you walk?" The patient and his or her family need to be told that acute pain is a warning sign and that rest is beneficial, but when pain continues for several months, there is no evidence that the pain means that something bad will happen.

Conditions at work or at home may be a source of stress, but identification of these factors does not always permit manipulation, though it is important to try. The physician should at least help the patient understand how tension created by his or her life situation may aggravate the pain and disability, and help the patient seek other ways of dealing with stress.

Psychoneurotic back discomfort is less effectively treated. Nevertheless, recognition allows problem solving and lays a basis for not doing more diagnostic tests in the pursuit of an elusive "diagnosis."

Low back pain may also be a manifestation, but usually not the only one, of depression. In this case, antidepressants are indicated. In a person with chronic pain, cause and effect are difficult to reconstruct, and an empirical therapeutic trial is indicated, even when the mechanism of the mood disorder is unclear.

The most difficult obstacle to altering a pattern of chronic back disability is the secondary gain from the illness. In occupational low-back injuries, for instance, provision of basic necessities such as food and shelter is only given for continued display of disability. If an individual has been disabled or unable to function effectively for more than a year, his or her life and the environment have molded around the patient. Patterns of dependence and interdependence, attitudes of friends and family, and employment have been set, and rehabilitation requires as much attention to the social milieu in which the person operates as it does to the patient.

In summary, the approach to the chronic back-pain patient is to:

1. Emphasize that pain is unlikely to change. Therefore, avoid the use of addicting medications.
2. Focus on function, not pain. Direct the patient's attention to stresses and coping behavior. Relaxation therapies and behavior modification may be options.
3. Treat depression if it is present.
4. Avoid patient dependency.
5. Limit opportunities for secondary gain at the outset.

REFERENCES

Aloia J, Cohn SH, Ostuni JA, Cane R, Ellis K: Prevention of involutional bone loss by exercise. Ann Intern Med 89:356–358, 1978.

Avioli LV: Osteoporosis: Pathogenesis and therapy. In Avioli LV, Krane SM (eds). *Metabolic Bone Disease*, Vol. 1. Academic Press, New York, 1977, p 301.

Bartelink DL: The role of abdominal pressure in relieving the pressure on the lumbar intervertebral discs. J Bone Joint Surg 398:718–725, 1957.

Beliveau P: A comparison between epidural anaesthesia with and without corticosteroid in the treatment of sciatica. Rheum Phys Med 11:40–43, 1971.

Brunarski DJ: Clinical trials of spinal manipulation: A critical appraisal and review of the literature. J Manipulative Physiol Ther 7:243–249, 1984.

Cady LD, Bischoff DP, O'Connell ER, et al.: Strength and fitness and subsequent back injuries in firefighters. J Occup Med 21:269–272, 1979.

Coxhead CE, Meade TW, Inskip H, North WRS, Troup JDG: Multicentre trail of physiotherapy in the management of sciatic symptoms. Lancet 1:1065–1068, 1981.

Crawshaw C, Frazer AM, Merriam WF, Mulholland RC, Webb JK: A comparison of surgery and chemonucleolysis in the treatment of sciatica. A prospective randomized trial. Spine 9:195–98, 1984.

Deyo RA: Conservative therapy for low back pain. JAMA 1983; 250:1057–1055.

Deyo RA, Diehl AK, Rosenthal M: How many days of bed rest for acute low back pain? A randomized clinical trial. N Engl J Med 1986; 315:1064–1070.

Dilke TFW, Barry HC, Grahame K: Extradural corticosteroid injection in the management of lumbar nerve root compression. Br Med J 2:635–637, 1973.

Doran DML, Newell DJ: Manipulation in treatment of low back pain: A multicentre study. Br Med J 2:161–164, 1975.

Finneson BE: Modulating effect of secondary gain on the low back pain syndrome. In *Advances in Pain Research and Therapy*, Vol. 1, Raven Press, New York, 1976, pp 949–952.

Fraser RD: Chymopapain for the treatment of intervertebral disc herniation: The final report of a double blind study. Spine 9:815–818, 1984.

Fraser RD: Chymopapain for the treatment of intervertebral disc herniation. Spine 7:608–612, 1982.

Fredrickson BE, Baker P, McHolick WJ, Yuan HA, Lubicky JP: The natural history of spondylolysis and spondylolisthesis. J Bone Joint Surg 66A:669–707, 1984.

Frymoyer JW: Back pain and sciatica. N Engl J Med 318:291–300, 1988.

Frymoyer JW, Hanley E, Howe J, Kuhlmann D, Matteri R: Disc excision and spine fusion in the management of lumbar disc disease. A minimum ten-year follow-up. Spine 3:1–6, 1978.

Gilbert JR, Taylor DW, Hildebrand A, Evans C: Clinical trial of common treatments for low back pain in family practice. Br Med J 291:791–794, 1985.

Gillstrom P, Ehrnberg A: Long-term results for autotraction in the treatment for lumbago and sciatica. An attempt to correlate clinical results with objective parameters. Arch Orthop Trauma Surg 104:294–298, 1985.

Gofton JP: Persistent low back pain and leg-length discrepancy. J Rheum 12:747–750, 1985.

Hadler NM: Low back pain. In Hadler NM (ed). *Medical Management of the Regional Musculoskeletal Disease*. Grune & Stratton Orlando, FL, 1984, pp 3–79.

Hahn TJ, Hahn BH: Osteopenia in patients with rheumatic diseases: Principles of diagnosis and therapy. Semin Arthritis Rheum 6:165–188, 1976.

Haldeman S: Spinal manipulative therapy. A status report. Clin Orthop 179:62–70, 1983.

Hall S, Bartleson JP, Onofrio BM, Baker HL, Okazaki H, O'Duffy JD: Lumbar spinal stenosis. Ann Intern Med 103:271–275, 1985.

Hammonds W, Brena S, Unikel I: Compensation for work-related injuries and rehabilitation of patients with chronic pain. South Med J 71:664–666, 1978.

Hoehler FK, Tobis JS, Buerger AA: Spinal manipulation for low back pain. JAMA 245:1835–1838, 1981.

Horsman A, Gallagher JC, Simpson M, Nordin BEC: Prospective trial of estrogen and calcium in post-menopausal women. Br Med J 2:789, 1977.

Jowsey J, Riggs BL, Kelly PJ, Hoffman DL: Effect of continued therapy with sodium fluoride, vitamin D and calcium in osteoprosis. Am J Med 53:43–49, 1972.

Kelman H: Epidural injection therapy for sciatic pain. Am J Surg 2:183–190, 1944.

Kendall PH, Jenkins JM: Exercise for backache: A double blind controlled trial. Physiotherapy 54:154–157, 1968.

Lankhorst GJ, Van DeStadt RJ, Vogelaar TW, Van DerKorst JK, Prevo AJH: The effect of Swedish back school in chronic idiopathic low back pain: A prospective controlled study. Scand J Rehabil Med 15:141–145, 1983.

Larsson U, Choler U, Lidstrom A, et al.: Auto-traction for treatment of lumbago-sciatica. A multicentre controlled investigation. Acta Orthop Scan 51:791–798, 1980.

Liang MH, Komaroff AL Roentgenograms in Primary care patients with acute low back pain: A cost-effectiveness analysis Arch Int Med 142:1108–1112, 1982.

Lidstrom A, Zachrisson M: Physical therapy on low back pain and sciatica. An attempt at evaluation. Scan J Rehab Med 2:37–42, 1970.

Lindsay R, Aitken JM, Anderson JB, Hart DM, MacDonald EB, Clarke AC: Long-term prevention of post-menopausal osteoporosis by estrogen. Lancet 1:1038, 1976.

McCulloch JA: Chemonucleolysis: Experience with 2000 cases. Clin Orthop 146:128–135, 1980.

Moffet JAK, Chase SM, Portek BS, Ennis JR: A controlled, prospective study to evaluate the effectiveness of a back school in the relief of chronic low back pain. Spine 11:120–122, 1986.

Mooney V, Cairns D, Robertson: A system for evaluating and treating chronic back disability. West J Med 124:370–376, 1976.

Mooney V, Robertson J: The facet syndrome. Clin Orthop 115:149–156, 1976.

Nachemson A: The lumbar spine: An orthopaedic challenge. Spine 1:59–71, 1976.

Nachemson A, Lindh M: Measurement of abdominal and back muscle strength with and without low back pain. Scand J Rehab Med 1:60–65, 1969.

Nachtigall LE, Nachtigall RH, Nachtigall RD, Beckman EM: Estrogen replacement therapy I: A 10-year prospective study in the relationship to osteoporosis. Obstet Gynecol 53:277–281, 1979.

Nakano KK: Sciatic nerve entrapment: The piriformis syndrome. J Musclo Med: 33–37, 1987.

Naylor A: The late results of laminectomy for lumbar disease prolapse. J Bone Joint Surg 56B:17–29, 1974.

Ottenbacher K, DiFabio RP: Efficacy of spinal manipulation/mobilization therapy. A meta-analysis. Spine 10:833–837, 1985.

Pal B, Mangion P, Hossain MA, Diffey BL: A controlled trial of continuous lumbar traction in the treatment of back pain and sciatica. Br J Rheumatol 25:181–183, 1986.

Payne RW, Sorenson EJ, Smalley TK, Brandt EN: Diazepam, mephrobamate, and placebo in musculoskeletal disorders. JAMA 188:229–232, 1964.

Pearce J, Moll JMH: Conservative treatment and natural history of acute lumbar disc lesions. J Neurol Neurosurg Psych 30:13–17, 1967.

Quinet RJ, Hadler NM: Diagnosis and treatment of backache. Semin Arthritis Rheum 8:261–287, 1979.

Recker RR, Saville RD, Hancy RP: Effects of estrogens and calcium carbonate on bone loss in post-menopausal women. Ann Intern Med 87:649–000, 1977.

Sarno JE: Psychosomatic backache. J Family Pract 5:353–357, 1977.

Sims-Williams H, Jayson MIV, Young SMS, Baddeley H, Collins E: Controlled trial of mobilization and manipulation for low back pain in hospital patients. Br Med J 2:1318–1320, 1979.

Sims-Williams H, Jayson MIV, Young SMS, Bradeley H, Collins E: Controlled trial of mobilization and manipulation for patients with low back pain in general practices. Br Med J 2:1338–1340, 1978.

Smythe HA: Nonarticular rheumatism and the fibrositis syndrome. In McCarthy DJ Jr (ed). *Arthritis and Allied Conditions.* 9th edition. Lea & Febiger, Philadelphia, 1989, pp 888–891.

Swezey RL: The modern thrust of manipulation and traction therapy. Semin Rheum Dis 12:321–331, 1983.

Verbiest H: Neurogenic intermittent claudication in cases with absolute and relative stenosis of the lumbar vertebral canal, in cases with narrow lumbar vertebral foramina, and in cases with both entities. Clin Neurosurg 20:204–214, 1973.

Weber H: Lumbar disc herniation. A controlled prospective study with 10 years of observation. Spine 2:131–140, 1983.

Weinstein J, Spratt KF, Lehmann T, McNeill T, Hejna W: Lumbar disc herniation. A comparison of the results of chemonucleolysis and open disectomy after ten years. J Bone Joint Surg 68A:43–54, 1986.

Weinstein JL: Idiopathic scoliosis: Natural history. Spine 11:780–783, 1986.

Wiesel SW, Cuckler JM, DeLuca F, Jones F, Zeids MS, Rothman RH: Acute low-back pain: An objective analysis of conservative therapy. Spine 5:324–330, 1980.

Wiesel SW, Sourmas N, Feffer HL, Citrin CM, Patronas N: Non-specific back pain. Spine 9:549–552, 1984.

5 Principles of Pain Management

Patients vary widely in their response to pain and, thus, management needs to be individualized. Some patients are stoical, others hysterical, others extremely fearful of pain's cause. Appropriate management involves an understanding of the pain's source and severity, the meaning of the pain to the individual, an understanding of the patient's personality, and structuring a regimen around this knowledge. Some patients need only an explanation of how the pain arose or how long it will last, others may need to be treated with analgesics.

ESTABLISHING THE CAUSE OF PAIN

The first priority is to establish the cause of the pain, because when specific therapy exists, it tends to be more effective than analgesia. Examples of relatively specific therapies are given in Table 5–1. In the absence of specific therapy, analgesics may be administered for pain relief: non-narcotic agents for mild, superficial pain; and narcotics for deep visceral or severe pain.

SEVERITY OF PAIN

Pain is a subjective experience, and thus the clinician can only estimate the intensity of a patient's pain and his pain threshold. Severe pain interferes with normal function or with sleep. The facial expression is a sensitive indicator of pain severity. A person who describes his pain in a theatrical, animated, or flat manner is unlikely to have severe pain. Differences in the expression of pain range from inhibition of expression on the one end to complete expression at the other. Expression of pain reflects, in part, social and cultural training.

The threshold of pain awareness and the ability to tolerate pain are decreased by anxiety, boredom, fatigue, coexisting illness, and protracted pain. Tolerance is increased by excitement, outside interests, group activities, work, diversion, and drugs. Recognizing that a patient in pain may have a low threshold alerts

TABLE 5–1. THE SPECIFIC TREATMENT OF PAIN

Type of Pain	"Specific" Therapy
Musculoskeletal	
Soft-tissue injury	Ice for acute injury, rest involved part
Bone pain — tumor	Radiation, indomethacin
osteomyelitis antibiotics	
Paget's disease	Calcitonin, diphosphonates
Neurogenic pain	
Tic douloureux	Carbamazepine, diphenylhydantoin
Post-herpetic neuralgia	" "
Phantom-limb pain	" "
Tabes dorsalis	" "
Trigeminal neuralgia	Electrocoagulation of the gasserian ganglion
Herniated disc with root compression	Laminectomy and decompression of nerve
Spinal stenosis	roots
Inflammatory	
Synovitis	Nonsteroidal, antiinflammatory agents Corticosteroids
Spondylitis	Indomethacin, phenylbutazone
Infection	Antibiotics
Abscess	Drainage, antibiotics
Bursitis	Local injection of corticosteroids
Ischemic pain	
Atherosclerotic disease	Vascular surgery
Emboli	Embolectomy
Vasculitis	Corticosteroids, immunosuppressive agents

one to deal with the factors responsible and to not overtreat with analgesics.

The meaning of the pain should be identified. Does the pain interfere with the person's normal activities? Does the patient want treatment, or does he want reassurance that nothing is serious and that it will go away? How do other family members or friends respond to the pain? What would happen in terms of improved function if the pain were entirely removed? When symptoms do not conform to known syndromes or there are no objective findings, psychological factors may be important, but the physician should not deny the existence of the symptom. These persons have real pain by any measure we choose; their suffering is real to them. Dr. E.A. Stead observed that narcotics are good drugs for pain but there is no drug for suffering. It follows that a cardinal feature of effective pain management is distinguishing between pain and suffering as clearly as possible.

ACUTE PAIN

Acute pain is of brief duration, temporary, often intermittent, and results from known mechanisms (migraine headaches, dental pain, postoperative pain, and childbirth). Anxiety and acute pain are intimately related. Acute pain produces anxiety, and anxiety may potentiate pain and reduce one's pain tolerance. Fear of not knowing what is wrong, what to expect, or when relief may come are commonly expressed by patients. Other patients feel helpless and unable to control their response to pain, because they fear that the pain will reach intolerable levels so that they will not be able to endure it. Other patients feel that pain is a signal that something is seriously wrong, for instance, a sign of cancer, and may react inappropriately to trivial symptoms because of their anxiety. The longer the pain lasts, the greater the anxiety.

Management of acute pain is strongly dependent on the physician's ability to reduce anxiety. Explaining how the pain is produced, what the treatment will be, the cause of the pain, and how long the pain will last is needed. The power of a simple explanation is illustrated in a classic study, which shows that telling patients what to expect during and after surgery resulted in shorter postoperative stays, on the average of 2.5 days shorter, than those of a control group that did not receive such an explanation.

A statement of what to expect does not need to be a precise probability statement, but an estimate of the course that allows the patient to cope with the symptoms, to make plans, and to undermine fantasies. Even if the estimates are not precise, the fact that the patient can act and make plans allows the individual to control his or her life, minimizing feelings of helplessness and loss of control.

If one "programs" the patient by saying, "If the pain is not better in x days, we'll get an x-ray or send you to a consultant," one can be sure that the symptom will *not* get better. Similarly, a negative suggestion such as, "Call me if the pain gets worse" will inevitably be fulfilled. Instead, say, "Call me if you need me" or "Call in x days."

Nonorganic (Psychogenic) Pain

Pain is not always associated with somatic disease. When no etiology is present, pain must be treated cautiously with careful follow-up. The diagnosis of psychogenic pain is suggested when the history or physical do not point to an organic cause, and pain is refractory to adequate analgesia. Patients may be oblivious to their psychological stress because the pain is at once a symptom and an escape from the feelings associated with the stress. The patient feels the pain physically, expects medical treatment, and may resent any suggestion that his pain is "in his head."

Some physicians feel obligated to treat only physical pathology, and when no "cause" is found, label the patient a "crock," or even react angrily by confronting the patient with the likelihood of psychogenic illness. On the other hand, if the physician accepts the patient's pain at face value and treats the symptom while continuing the search for an organic source, the symptoms are likely to worsen. After an initial response, the patient returns with worse pain, and the physician will increase the intensity of the diagnostic procedures to look for a physical origin, which reinforces the misperception that the problem is organic.

The rule-out style of diagnosis before a psychological cause creates needless expense and delay in providing useful treatment; and worse yet, it reinforces noncoping pain behavior. The manner in which the diagnosis of psychogenic pain is presented to the patient is critical in the patient's acceptance of the diagnosis. One must not imply that the pain is "all in the head" or dismiss all physical basis for the complaint. Hostility may result, and the patient may go away to someone who "will take care of him" or who will take him seriously.

The physician should acknowledge that the suffering is real, that there is no question of the patient faking, or that he is crazy. Explain how emotions can cause or intensify pain. This face-saving maneuver allows the patient to keep the symptoms but at the same time provides a basis for dealing with them.

In the process of discussing emotional problems, the patient may focus less on the pain and more and more on areas of conflict in living. If a psychiatric diagnosis of neurosis such as depression or anxiety is made, specific psychopharmacy may be useful.

Therapeutic objectives should emphasize activity rather than symptoms. Instead of asking, "How are you?" or "How do you feel?" ask about activity, "What did you do yesterday?" or "How much have you been able to do?" or "How far can you walk?" The patient and the family need to understand that pain is a warning sign and that rest is beneficial with acute pain, but that chronic pain continuing unchanged has no prognostic meaning. This important point in management is discussed in detail in the section on treatment of psychogenic back pain.

PAIN TREATMENT

Pain Medication

People's attitudes toward pain medication are unpredictable. Some feel that since analgesics are freely available they should be taken to relieve any unpleasant sensation, while others take the view that medications are "unnatural." Many would prefer to experience moderate pain, if it is not too severe or prolonged, rather than the peculiar, unpleasant sensations they get from taking medication. About one-third of postoperative patients say that the severity of their pain took them by surprise and some patients were resentful that they had not been warned that such pain might occur.

Regular administration of analgesics prevents pain from increasing in intensity, as so often happens when medications are taken on an as-needed basis. Unfortunately, administering analgesics as needed also pairs the symptom (pain) with the reinforcement (medication) — a potent method of conditioning, which may contribute to pain behavior and dependence on medications. For example, the risk of oral narcotic addiction rises to about double the baseline risk when an "as needed" regimen is substituted for a rigid schedule.

If the physician treats pain inadequately, the patient may need to ask for stronger medication or report worsened symptoms to get pain relief, which may also contribute to pain behavior. Physicians often use inadequate doses of narcotic analgesia in patients with acute pain for fear of addiction because of inaccurate knowledge about the addictive potential of narcotics.

Pain medication will be "more effective" if the physician explains the purpose and what to expect. Possible side effects and toxicity should also be

TABLE 5–2. TREATING ACUTE PAIN TO PREVENT CHRONIC PAIN

1. Give pain medication for a specified period.
2. Give the patient a specifically graded program to return to full activity.
3. Use modalities such as rest, heat, ice, or appliances whenever possible to relieve muscculoskeletal pain.
4. Set return visits at fixed time intervals so the patient does not need to have pain to justify a visit.
5. Get history of drug and alcohol use before prescribing new medications.
6. Make sure the dose of analgesic is effective for pain relief before giving a second, potentiating agent for sedation.
7. Taper pain medications to prevent a flare-up of pain on abrupt withdrawal.

mentioned so that the patient will not discontinue the medication unnecessarily. Analgesics should be prescribed for a fixed period with instructions to taper the medication slowly. Follow-up is needed to ensure that the episode of pain has resolved.

Some patients who need analgesics will be concerned about becoming addicted. This is a healthy and legitimate concern, which should be addressed directly. Both habituation and addiction are less likely to occur if medications are given on a regular schedule without increasing the dose for small changes in the pain level.

The health care provider is in a strategic position to make things worse than they are and to facilitate dependencies or unrealistic expectations. Successful management of an acute pain will result in healthy attitudes and behaviors when pain is experienced in the future. The principles outlined are summarized in Table 5–2.

Acute pain can be managed effectively with non-narcotic analgesics. Aspirin is the first choice. Newer pain medications and combinations of analgesics have added little, except novelty and expense. Codeine, a narcotic with low abuse liability is an inexpensive and underutilized pain medication. In the sections that follow, the clinical pharmacology of commonly used analgesics will be summarized.

Salicylates and salicylate equivalents

Salicylates are the oldest and most commonly used of the analgesic and anti-inflammatory agents. Although a number of salicylic acid derivatives have been developed, acetylsalicylate (aspirin) is superior in both its antiinflammatory and its analgesic effects to other salicylate derivatives. In terms of its analgesic effect, double-blind, crossover studies comparing aspirin to equal doses of mefenamic acid, pentazocine, acetaminophen, phenacetin, and codeine show it to be superior to these agents and placebo.

Tinnitus is an early and reliable sign of salicylate toxicity in adults. In young adults, tinnitus occurs in the range of 20 to 30 mg%, which corresponds to an antiinflammatory serum level. However, tinnitus is an unreliable symptom of toxicity in the very young, the very old, and people with hearing loss. In these clinical settings, a determination of the serum salicylate level is the only way to titrate the dose.

High-dose aspirin commonly causes gastric discomfort, nausea, anorexia, and deafness. The damaging effect of aspirin on the gastric mucosa is thought to be a direct and systemic one. Salicylate, in its un-ionized form, readily crosses cell membranes. In an acid environment in the stomach, un-ionized salicylate passes freely inside the mucosal cells, but becomes ionized at the intracellular pH and is only slowly transported out of the cell. Thus, high concentrations accumulate intracellularly and interfere with normal mechanisms that protect the mucosa against damage by acid. Aspirin and other nonsteroidal antiinflammatory agents also inhibit endogeneous prostaglandins, which also contribute to gastric mucosal damage.

Dilution of the drug with food or fluid, buffering of the aspirin, and rapid complete dispersion of the tablet substantially reduce the potential for gastric irritation. Plain aspirin tablets disintegrate in the stomach and dissolve primarily in the small intestine; it is the dissolution rate that determines the rate of absorption into the bloodstream. Theoretically, some manufactured tablets might be so tightly packed that they are not readily dissolved or they may crumble before use. Although these differences between tablets could have clinical consequences, it has never been demonstrated that one brand of plain aspirin is superior to another in terms of its analgesic effect.

Buffers increase pH at the surface of aspirin particles, but in the amounts present in most formulations, buffers do not significantly decrease gastric acidity. Food or a full glass of water with each dose is as good a buffer as the amount of antacid in most buffered aspirin tablets. Leonards and Levy found less gastrointestinal bleeding with buffered tablets, but it has never been established in patients with painful conditions that buffered aspirin results in a difference in the time of onset of analgesia, the duration or degree of pain relief, or the incidence of gastrointestinal distress. Peak serum levels will be achieved more rapidly when aspirin is in solution than when a tablet must first dissolve, but there is no good evidence that buffered solutions produce more rapid or more effective analgesia than plain or buffered aspirin tablets. Alka-Selzer®, an effervescent formulation of aspirin, contains a higher content of buffering agents than Bufferin® or other buffered aspirin tablets. It is an effective way of taking single doses of aspirin and it causes less gastrointestinal bleeding than the plain or buffered aspirin tablets. However, the high content of sodium (516 mg/tablet) and bicarbonate and its relatively high cost, make Alka-Selzer® less useful than other formulations of aspirin for long-term use.

Time-released aspirin contains small encapsulated particles of the drug bound together in a tablet. Absorption of these aspirin preparations is slightly delayed and prolonged. Enteric-coated aspirin tablets have special coats that delay absorption without any loss in physiological ability. These preparations may be variably absorbed, but this point is not clinically significant when the medication is used regularly. Nonacetylated salicylates produce less gastritis and do not interfere with platelet adhesiveness, can be used in aspirin allergy, and include choline salicylate, salsalate, and choline magnesium salicylate.

Many aspirin formulations include other drugs such as phenacetin, salicylamide, acetaminophen, caffeine, or antihistamines. The specific combinations often vary within a given brand name from year to year. Such combinations have never been proven more effective than aspirin alone and may only cause a higher incidence of adverse effects.

The regular ingestion of most forms of salicylate is associated with blood loss in the gastrointestinal tract, and may be, in some rare cases, sufficient to cause hypochromic anemia. Aspirin increases the bleeding time but is clinically unimportant in the majority of patients. Fifty percent to 80% of salicylate in the serum is bound to albumin. Drugs that may be displaced from protein binding by salicylate, and therefore potentiated, include coumadin, diphenylhydantoin, the oral hypoglycemic agents, phenylbutazone, and some hormones. The total serum level of hormones that are protein bound is reduced in patients taking aspirin, but active free hormone is maintained by normal control mechanisms and endocrine dysfunction does not occur. Minor side effects in patients given large doses of aspirin include drowsiness, increased sweating, and constipation.

Serious hypersensitivity to aspirin in the form of bronchospasm and hypotension is rare. Minor manifestations such as swelling of the nasal mucosa and nasal polyps are more common. In patients with systemic lupus erythematosus, juvenile rheumatoid arthritis, rheumatoid arthritis, and in occasional normal persons, abnormalities of liver function can be detected; the clinical significance of abnormal liver function tests in normal individuals is unknown. Aspirin is not teratogenic, but there is a suggestion that regular aspirin takers during pregnancy have an increased incidence of anemia, antipartum and postpartum hemorrage, prolonged gestation, complicated deliveries, and perinatal mortality when compared with nontakers.

Acetaminophen

Acetaminophen has been used as an analgesic and antipyretic agent for over 80 years. In the United States, it is marketed under approximately 50 brand names and in almost 200 proprietary combinations with other drugs.

Acetaminophen has analgesic and antipyretic effects similar to those of aspirin, but has little antiinflammatory action. In two well-designed studies of postpartum pain, 600 mg of acetaminophen was equal in analgesic effectiveness to 600 mg of aspirin and was much superior to placebo. In pain due to cancer, 600 mg of acetaminophen and 600 or 1200 mg of aspirin were significantly superior to placebo, but not significantly different from one another; the time to onset of pain relief was similar. A recent study using several criteria of pain relief effectiveness in cancer patients confirmed that there is no significant difference between acetaminophen and aspirin in 650 mg doses and that both were significantly superior to placebo. The antipyretic effects of aspirin and acetaminophen are comparable in adults and children.

Acetaminophen does not cause gastric irritation, erosions, or gastrointestinal bleeding. It does not interfere with platelet function, interact with oral anticoagulants, nor alter uric acid excretion. Acetaminophen is, therefore, often used for patients who are intolerant of aspirin and for patients with bleeding disorders or those taking oral anticoagulants.

Hypersensitivity reactions to acetaminophen are very uncommon. Although acetaminophen has been weakly implicated in the syndrome of analgesic nephropathy, and chronic interstitial nephritis, the cause of this syndrome is far from established. Nephropathy has not been reported in patients using only acetaminophen.

Hepatotoxicity may result from chronic consumption of moderate doses of acetaminophen. Hepatic central lobular necrosis results from a single overdose of 10 g and death from 25 g. Evidence of damage can be seen 24 to 48 hours after an overdose of acetaminophen but may not plateau until 4 to 6 days after ingestion. In severely intoxicated patients, hepatic involvement may progress to encephalopathy, coma, and death within a few days.

The usual oral dose of acetaminophen is 325 to 650 mg for adults. The dose is repeated every 3 to 4 hours as necessary, and if the dose of 650 mg is ineffective, it is unlikely that higher doses will afford more relief. The total daily dose of acetaminophen should not exceed 3 g in adults or 1.2 g in a child. With impairment of hepatic function, lower doses should be given.

The maximal analgesic dose of acetaminophen has not been determined. Single doses of 650 mg appear to be clearly more effective than doses around 300 mg, and 1 g may provide somewhat more relief than 650 mg, but the difference is marginal. However, no amount of the drug will adequately relieve severe pain of any origin.

Codeine

Orally, a dose of 32 mg of codeine is equipotent to 600 mg of aspirin. When these two drugs are combined, there is a significant synergistic effect. Doses ranging from 15 to 30 mg orally are effective in suppressing the frequency of pathological cough. The abuse potential of codeine is much lower than that of morphine and other narcotics. It is inexpensive and is usually free of side effects. An occasional patient may get "snowed" or "feel spacey" with this medication, however.

Propoxyphene

Propoxyphene hydrochloride (Darvon®) is a narcotic analgesic that is structurally related to methadone. Its potency is probably less than that of aspirin and codeine, but it is better tolerated than codeine. Side effects such as nausea, vomiting, epigastric distress, dizziness, drowsiness, pruritus, and skin rashes are minimal. The usual dosage is 65 mg every 4 to 6 hours.

Antiinflammatory agents (Table 5–3)

To aspirin and formulations of aspirin are added to a long list of nonsteroidal antiinflammatory drugs (NSAIDs) that affect inflammation. As a generalization, all NSAIDs block, to varying degrees, enzymes along the arachadonic acid

TABLE 5–3. NONSTEROIDAL ANTIINFLAMMATORY DRUGS (NSAIDS)*

Salicylates	**Proprionic Acid Derivatives**
Aspirin Diflunisal (Dolobid)	Ibuprofen (Motrin, Bufren, Advil, Nuprin) Naproxen (Naprosyn) Fenoprofen (Nalfon, Fenopron) Ketoprofen (Alrheuma, Orudis)
Nonacetylated salicylates	
Magnesium choline salicylate (Disalcid) Salasate (Trilisate) Choline salicylate (Arthropan)	
Indoles	**Phenylacetic Acid Deriatives**
Indomethacin (Indocin, Indocid) Sulindac (Clinoril) Tolmetin (Tolectin)	Diclofenac (Voltaren) **Oxicams** Piroxicam (Feldene)
Pyrazoles	**Fenamates**
Phenylbutazone (Butazolidin) Oxyphenbutazone (Tanderil)	Mefenamic acid (Ponstel) Meclofenamate sodium (Meclomen)

* Common brand names are in parentheses.

pathway, even though one may have more specific effects on one aspect of the pathway than the other. Currently there are over 20 licensed NSAIDs in the United States. The world over, there are over 200 NSAIDs used.

NSAIDs are used in postoperative pain, premenstrual syndrome, headache, and in inflammatory arthritis.

All NSAIDs have been tested in clinical trials against aspirin in antiinflammatory doses, and as a rule, they produce less gastrointestinal bleeding and other side effects (although they occur) and require far fewer tablets to achieve an antiinflammatory effect. In exchange for these advantages, the patient pays more and is exposed to other side effects, which include rash, cognitive disturbances, and a number of renal syndromes that have not been seen clinically with aspirin. In addition, phenylbutazone may cause rare cases of fatal aplastic anemia or agranulocytosis.

In this setting, we are conservative. This story leads one to follow the adage ascribed to Russell Cecil, which roughly paraphrased is: Prescribe drugs that have been on the market for a year or less only to a dying patient; for 5 years to other patients; for 10 years to family members; and for 20 years or more to oneself.

Some patients do better on one NSAID than another. Whether this is chance, the natural history of the disease, or actual differences in individual responsiveness or differences between NSAIDs is not known. One logical possibility that applies to ibuprofen (which has an active and an inactive steroisomer) and to sulindac, is that there are differences in patients' abilities to convert the drug between active and inactive forms. Some patients also believe that they become resistant to particular initially effective drugs over time. This phenomenon is not understood in even a rudimentary way. In chronic disease, during flares or over a prolonged course, it is inevitable that the patient or the doctor will want to try something different. One rational approach is to learn one drug from each class. Table 5–3 provides a classification of NSAIDs by family of drugs. Most NSAIDs interfere with platelet function, but clinically important bleeding is rare. The nonsalicylate NSAIDs' effects on platelets are relatively short lived, and after stopping the dose, platelet functional deficits are gone by 48 hours. Salicylates, with the exception of the nonacetylated salicylates, interfere with platelet aggregation for up to 7 to 10 days after the dose has stopped due to irreversible inhibition of cyclooxygenase.

The NSAIDs, with the exception of salicylates, may cause renal syndromes, which include acute renal insufficiency, nephrotic syndrome, interstitial nephritis, and papillary necrosis. NSAIDs, because of their affect on renal blood flow, can cause fluid retention and diminished salt excretion. Hemodynamic renal toxicity is more likely in patients with underlying renal disease, particularly in individuals with renal vascular disease or in people with diminished intravascular volume such as occurs in chronic diuretic therapy, congestive heart failure, cirrhosis, and nephrosis. Acute renal failure from NSAIDs occurs anywhere from 2 weeks to 18 months after starting the agent, and for this period laboratory monitoring with a urine analysis and serum creatinine is suggested.

Some NSAIDs cause blood dyscrasias. Agranulocytosis or aplastic anemia has been reported with indomethacin, ibuprofen, fenaprofen, naprosyn, tolmetin, parixocam, sulindac, and phenylbutazone; and the time of onset after starting NSAIDs is unpredicable. However, blood dyscrasias are rare and are likely to be idiosyncratic events. One should have a low threshold for getting a blood count in patients on NSAIDs, particularly if there are symptoms that suggests infection, leukopenia, and anemia, such as mouth sores, fever, and fatigue.

A variety of NSAIDs cause mild elevations in liver enzymes and occasionally cholestatic hepatitis. Again, these are rare and liver function tests are not usually obtained in the absence of symptoms in patients taking NSAIDs other than diclofenac. A reduced ability to metabolize drugs by the liver or the kidney make the elderly vulnerable to drug toxicity, and such patients should be started on reduced doses and followed regularly.

Phenylbutazone

Phenylbutazone is a potent antiinflammatory drug, but because of its potential serious toxicity, its routine use for self-limited illnesses should be restricted. It is the impression of many clinicians that the drug is frequently beneficial in the treatment of bursitis, tendinitis, and acute tenosynovitis. Some patients with spondylo-arthropathies respond to phenylbutazone but not to other NSAIDs.

The metabolism of the drug occurs principally through an inducible liver enzyme, which explains the wide individual variation in the duration of action. Toxic effects from phenylbutazone occur abruptly, or may be related to both the dose and duration of treatment. Death from bone marrow suppression occurs in 1 in 50,000 patients. Other complications include gastrointestinal ulceration, hepatitis, and renal failure. Sodium retention is frequently encountered, but is usually only significant in those patients with poor cardiac reserve.

Phenylbutazone strongly inhibits the binding of some drugs to serum and tissue proteins, and potentiates their effects. Coumadin and the oral hypoglycemic agents are such examples. Other drugs are rendered less effective because phenylbutazone stimulates the cytochrome enzyme system, which is involved in its own metabolism and the oxidation of other drugs, including phenobarbital, diphenylhydantoin, tolbutamide, and digitoxin.

Indomethacin

Indomethacin is a potent antiinflammatory drug but has little analgesic effect. Indomethacin is beneficial in the treatment of bursitis, tendinitis, and acute tenosynovitis, but formal studies are lacking. In a variety of soft-tissue injuries, sprains, and strains, indomethacin in a dose of 50 mg, three times daily, was not significantly different from placebo in British soccer players. There was no difference between the treated and the control group in terms of pain, swelling, and the duration of disability after injury.

In osteoarthritis, indomethacin is superior to placebo, as judged by patient preference, pain on walking, pain at rest, and the range of hip movement, but indomethacin causes twice as many side effects as placebo.

However, in hospitalized patients with osteoarthritis, 3.9 g of aspirin compared to 150 mg of indomethacin for 10 days, with a crossover the second 10 days, showed no significant differences in subjective or objective criteria in improvement between indomethacin and aspirin. The lack of difference may have been because both groups were hospitalized and bed rested. In any case, indomethacin is useful in the management of degenerative joint disease of the hip and knee. Although pain and mobility in hip disease may improve, the anatomical progression of the disease is not slowed.

The maximum tolerated doses of indomethacin are in the range of 100–200 mg per day. Side effects are frequent and occur in about one third of all patients, and especially in older age groups. Indomethacin is ulcerogenic and should be given with food to reduce gastric irritation. Central nervous system effects preclude its use in 30% to 50% of patients. Most of these effects are mild and consist of headaches and vague affective syndromes ranging from depression to mild hallucinations. Unsteadiness of gait or frank ataxia has been reported in some long-term users. Although it is claimed that these side effects may be minimized by gradual increases of medication to therapeutic levels, this strategy is not always successful.

Physical Modalities

Numerous physical modalities are used in the treatment of patients with arthritis and musculoskeletal complaints, and include techniques of delivering heat, cold, or physical stimulation to soft tissue. The physiological bases of these are not well understood, but patients find relief; and, therefore, it is useful to be aware of the possibilities. Another advantage of these modalities is that they involve patients actively in their therapy.

There is no evidence that heat is preferable to cold for arthritis and musculoskeletal complaints. In general, acute symptoms of sprains and strains are best treated by cold application. Chronic soft-tissue pain or muscle spasm respond better to heat, preferably moist heat. It is best to apply this general sequence but to individualize it for each patient.

Heat may be applied with friction massage, ultrasound, hydroculator packs, and hot packs generated by chemical reaction. Paraffin, diathermy, and infrared are techniques that have become less popular.

Cold is applied mainly by the use of ice packs and sometimes a cooling spray, ethyl chloride. Inexpensive ways of applying cold include using a large bag of frozen peas or freezing ice in a paper cup with a popsicle stick.

Massage is useful for pains originating from muscle, but why it works or whether it works in specific clinical situations are both untested.

Hydrotherapy is therapeutic exercise done in water, be it a heated pool, whirlpool, or Hubbard tank. Muscle tension appears to be reduced and painful joints can be manipulated or moved without the stress (and pain) produced by weight bearing.

Electrical stimulation for pain relief is most commonly given by TENS (transcutaneous electrical nerve stimulation), which involves high-frequency, low-amplitude impulses delivered through paste by skin electodes over the painful area. TENS may act through overloading the pain afferent pathways (pain-gating theory). Some patients with chronic musculoskeletal pain respond remarkably well to transcutaneous nerve stimulation, and it is our impression that these patients are more likely to have radicular nerve pain. They often experience temporary relief of pain after electromyography or nerve conduction study.

Another electrical therapy is neuroprobe, in which points of low electrical resistence are found on the skin using an electrode and then a relatively painful electrical impulse is delivered through the point. These points seem to correspond to traditional acupuncture points.

Exercise Prescriptions

Painful joints can lose functional capacity from synovitis, soft-tissue contractures, and disuse muscle atrophy. Restricting normal joint motion in normal persons will lead to a diminished range of motion, sometimes in as early as 7 to 10 days, and muscles not used can atrophy over the same period. For conditions in which the joint is immobilized for prolonged periods, attention should be given to maintaining flexibility and muscle strength. If a patient is elderly or is not used to physical activity, supervised therapy may be helpful. Important examples of such prevention procedures are Codman exercises for people with shoulder problems and quadriceps strengthening for people with knee problems. These have been detailed in Chapters 2 and 3.

For patients with chronic polyarthritis, there needs to be a balance of resting the involved joints to avoid aggravating synovitis, but also exercise to maintain the range of motion and muscle strength. An individualized program may be beyond the experience of the physician and may require consultation from those sophisticated in longitudinal assessment and management of such patients. Aside from specific exercises for involved joints, patients with chronic illnesses become deconditioned, and this can contribute to the sense of a lack of well-being, diminished endurance, and fatigue. Contrary to popular teaching, patients with chronic arthritis and other chronic illnesses may exercise to improve their aerobic capacity. This is usually well tolerated, does not make the underlying disease flare up (when prescribed with supervision), and can improve the quality of their existence.

Chiropracty is based on the unproven idea that the alignment of the vertebrae is at the root of many musculoskeletal pains. Sometimes chiropracty may work remarkably well, but the relief is usually short lived. Chiropracty can be used as an ancillary measure as long as one is sure that the manipulations will not cause harm (such as in a C1-C2 subluxation of the neck causing neck pain in a patient with rheumatoid synovitis or the patient with ankylosing spondylitis with calcified spinal ligaments). Radiographs of the area involved are advisable before treatment is begun.

Steroid Joint Injections

Local injections of steroids and/or lidocaine can make an important contribution to symptomatic management in many forms of arthritis and soft-tissue rheumatism. Corticosteroids given intraarticularly can reduce both cartilage synthesis and destruction of cartilage matrix by metalloproteases released into joint fluid in fulminant inflammatory states. Because steroids can delay healing, and lidocaine can make a joint "anesthetic," more than four injections in a single site during a year or more than six intraarticular injections during the lifetime of a joint are not recommended.

Equipment

The rule is to use the smallest needle that will do the job. For injection only, the smallest needle is 25 gauge. For aspiration of joint fluid, the smallest effective needle bore is 22 gauge. If the fluid is particularly thick, an 18-gauge needle will be required. An 18-gauge needle requires local anesthesia, whereas with the other gauge needles, the pain of giving local anesthesia is almost as bad as putting the needle in. Local anesthesia may be provided by distraction, ice, ethyl chloride spray, and intradermal Xylocaine® (1%) without epinephrine. Ethyl chloride spray is the quickest.

Many steroid preparations are available for intraarticular or soft-tissue injections. These include Depo-Medrol®, Celestone®, and Aristospan®. None carries a large advantage despite theoretical and in-vitro evidence that the solutions have differences in particle size, solubility, duration of action, and antiinflammatory potency. Triamcinolone acetomide (Kenalog®) and methylprednisolone (Depomedrol®) give the smallest incidences of facial flushing (20%) and postinjection flare when injected in muscle. For large joints such as the shoulder, the subdeltoid bursa, the trochanteric bursa, and the knee, 40 mg of Depomedrol or its equivalent is used. For smaller joints of the hands and feet or for other bursae, 20 mg of Depomedrol is adequate.

Lidocaine (xylocaine) can be added to the steroid. The amount varies from 1 to 2 ccs of Xylocaine 1% *without* epinephrine and depends on whether a large volume can be accepted by the joint or whether a large volume is required (i.e., for adhesive capsulitis). The epinephrine-containing lidocaine is avoided because of the small risk of causing an arrhythmia. An advantage of giving Xylocaine with steroid is that one gets a prompt notion of whether the injection is in the right place. An occasional patient will benefit despite not getting an immediate response from the Xylocaine, perhaps due to a systemic effect from an intra-articular or periarticular injection of steroid.

Almost any joint can be injected, but for someone not accustomed to the procedure we would advise restricting oneself to injecting the subdeltoid bursae or the shoulder joint proper, the olecranon bursa, the anserine and other bursae of the knee joint, the trochanteric bursa, and the true ankle joint. The inexperienced should avoid injecting carpel tunnel problems, joints of the hand, the hip joint, and other small joints of the feet.

Some points to remember are:

1. If there is any resistance in an intraarticular injection, stop.
2. In a tendon sheath injection, if there is resistance of any sort, redirect the needle. A true tendon sheath injection will distend the tendon sheath without resistance and should be visible as the sheath fills.
3. When placing the needle, stretch the skin tautly and inject perpendicular to the skin. Once through, advance slowly and redirect as needed.
4. Use new bottles of steroid and Xylocaine for each injection where possible.

The most feared complication of injection or aspiration is infection. This is rare, fortunately, when proper aseptic technique is used. Occasionally, patients will have an inflammatory response to an injection, which may be due to steroid crystals from the injection itself, a few hours after. This can be treated prophylactically by an NSAID given for several days afterwards and with ice to the area. Another complication is tendon rupture, which can occur if steroid is injected directly into a tendon. This is exceedingly rare and is avoided by never continuing with an injection if there is any resistance and never injecting a tendon of a weight-bearing joint such as the Achilles tendon. Multiple injections into a weight-bearing joint can cause a Charcot-like joint in 1% to 4% of cases.

Psychosocial Management

Patients with chronic disease need to cope with their symptoms and disabilities for life and through the ups and downs of their disease. Health care providers are partners with the patient in learning about the disease and helping them to adapt. Patients go through similar problems, and this chapter outlines common areas of concern and first principles of management.

The goal of psychosocial management is to equip patients with the information, attitudes, and coping skills that will allow them to function maximally. Indeed, patients with a chronic illness should become their own physicians for self-monitoring and, to some extent, adjustment of regimens, along with the physician.

For the rheumatic diseases discussed in Part 2 of this book, it is assumed that the primary care physician will be working with a specialist. However, since the primary physician is the physician of first contact and knows the patient best, many day-to-day problems will be brought to his or her attention for resolution. Many organizations devoted to rheumatic disorders provide important moral support to patients. These include the Arthritis Foundation, the SLE Foundation, the Ankylosing Spondylitis Society, and the Scleroderma Foundation. In some areas, the local chapter of the Arthritis Foundation is the umbrella organization for rheumatic diseases and can be the point of first referral for community resources. Social workers, physical and occupational therapists, and vocational counselors are valuable allies in conditions with multiple impacts, and the patient should be referred when appropriate.

The common problems of coping center around the following major issues: uncertainty, fatigue, depression, and compliance.

Uncertainty of diagnosis/prognosis

Uncertainty of either diagnosis or prognosis is common in lupus and other inflammatory rheumatic disorders in which symptoms may wax and wane, and in which vague symptoms may not be diagnosable. The patient is not able to predict from day to day or even week to week whether he or she will be the same, worse, or better. This ambiguity can lead to anxiety and preoccupation with somatic complaints.

A common phenomena in the early course of lupus is the tendency to attribute all symptoms to the lupus. The physician can help by equipping patients with some guidelines for self-monitoring so that they can develop confidence in their own ability to recognize a flare. Uncertainty, however, is contagious and it is frequently the physican who has no idea whether the patient is actually going to get worse.

The anxiety and fear that come with learning of a bad or chronic diagnosis or when a patient is "in flare" can be neutralized somewhat by discussing what to expect and what to look for in concrete terms, by a physician who is comfortable with uncertainty, by a physician who expresses commitment to helping the patient regardless of whether the symptoms can be irradicated, and by an explicit plan of action that is outlined in concrete terms. Uncertainty can also be diffused by a thorough approach and by being available.

Only a small percentage of the chronic rheumatic disorders discussed have an unrelenting course, and one can be guardedly optimistic. The other points to get across to the patient are that there is a plan and that the disease can be controlled, even if not actually cured. Most patients with chronic illness, in fact, manage and adapt very well.

Patients will undoubtedly seek other sources of information. This search, however, can cause as many problems as it helps. Most of the formal medical literature presents the experience of referral patients and thus the very worst or complicated cases. It would be well to correct these impressions. Ask the individual whether he or she has any personal experience or has read anything about the condition in order to see what emotional content issues forth.

Fatigue

Fatigue is a prominent and common symptom with many chronic illnesses. It may be due to anemia, depression, disease activity, medications used in treating rheumatic illnesses such as steroids, an associated illness, disturbed sleep and/or night pain, and deconditioning from inactivity or prescribed rest. Fatigue, though impairing the quality of life and function, is usually not addressed as a separate clinical problem because it is assumed to be inevitable, from depression, or untreatable.

Validate the patient's concern. Even in the absence of a specific cause, it is possible to help the patient. In disease flares, patients should rest when they are tired, rest involved joints, and nap. Fatigue is, in part, secondary to deconditioning, and a supervised program of 8 to 10 weeks of aerobic exercise will improve the way a deconditioned person feels. Such a program does not appear to make quiescent synovitis worse.

In contrast, adjustments may be needed at work, leisure activities, and in self-care when the disease is active. A working patient with arthritis may hide problems to avoid losing a job. Some employers resent direct interference or take it out on the patient if there are too many demands. To provide hope, the doctor himself must be able to accept disaster, be available, and communicate frankly and directly, even when no immediate solutions or possibility of amelioration exist. As one patient put it, "It's just the fact that you don't look away when I tell you this."

What a patient needs from a relationship with the doctor varies and changes. For example, there may be periods when the patient wants to negotiate and control medical care and other times, for example, during a flare, when a patient may want to be told what to do and to be dependent. Over the long run, the physician who can sense these changes and who is adaptable will have the most success in caring for chronic illnesses and patients.

Depression

Some depression is inevitable, but when the patient appears to have loss of function out of proportion to the objective impairment or has vegetative symptoms such as sleep disturbance, fatigue, and weight loss, then depression and psychosocial causes should be considered. A differential includes the following: lack of social support, particularly within the family; lack of identification with a single physician; and a sense of helplessness resulting from lack of knowledge of the disease.

Compliance

Nonadherence to medication or noncompliance is a symptom requiring diagnosis. If the patient is not made to feel guilty and states he or she missed some medication, cannot remember the medication, or has difficulty taking the medicine, noncompliance is likely, but doctors are notoriously inaccurate in assessing compliance. The reasons why patients (even doctor patients) do not follow advice range from the mundane to the subtle, and going through the major groups is needed to begin. The physician's advice might not have been heard, understood, remembered, or believed, or the prescription may have run out or been lost. The treatment may have been worse than the pain and may have caused unacceptable side effects or even toxicity. The medication may have been too expensive or too inconvenient in dosing schedule.

REFERENCES

Abramson SB, Weissman G: The mechanisms of action of nonsteroidal antiinflammatory drugs. Arthritis Rheum 32:1–9, 1989.

Liang MH: Psychosocial aspects of rheumatic disorders. In Kelley WH, Harris T, Ruddy S, Sledge CB (eds). *Textbook of Rheumatology*. Saunders, Philadelphia, WB 1989, pp 611–620.

Schoen RT: Mechanisms of nonsteroidal antiinflammatory drug-induced gastric damage. Am J Med 86:449–458, 1989.

TWO

Rheumatic disorders

6

Osteoarthritis

Osteoarthritis (also called osteoarthrosis and hypertropic or degenerative joint disease) is the most common form of arthritis. Radiographically it is seen in virtually all patients over the age of 50, but only a portion are symptomatic. In the United States, osteoarthritis is second only to cardiac disease as a cause of permanent incapacity in persons over the age of 50.

Osteoarthritis is generally categorized into primary osteoarthritis or secondary osteoarthritis. Primary osteoarthritis is the most common and is defined by the absence of any known predisposing factor, while secondary osteoarthritis occurs as the result of an underlying condition (Table 6–1). Primary osteoarthritis accounts for 90% of patients with osteoarthritis in unselected practices. The most commonly involved joints are the distal interphalangeal and the proximal interphalangeal joints of the fingers, the hip, the knee, the first metatars a phalangeal joint, and the cervical and lumbosacral spine. Some degenerative change in articular cartilage is universal with increasing age, but the onset, rate of progression, and severity vary greatly. If a joint is malaligned or has been traumatized or inflamed, changes appear more rapidly. Secondary osteoarthritis results from mechanical incongruity and/or cartilage destruction, which may be caused by congenital defects, joint infection or inflammation, trauma, or metabolic disease.

CLINICAL PRESENTATION

The most common presenting symptoms in patients with osteoarthritis are pain, stiffness, joint enlargement, and limitation of joint motion. The pain of osteoarthritis begins insidiously. Initially, patients describe an aching discomfort after use. Morning stiffness or stiffness after prolonged immobility generally lasts less than 30 minutes. Early in the course, joint pain occurs after vigorous activity, but with progression of cartilage damage, pain may occur after even minimal activity, and eventually even at rest. For most patients with early osteoarthritis,

TABLE 6–1. CLASSIFICATION OF OSTEOARTHROSES

Primary — 90%

Secondary — 10%

Previous Injury/Inflammation
Infectious arthritis
Inflammatory agent
Hemiarthrosis
Torn menisci, s/p menisectomy

Abnormal Cartilage
Acaptonuria
Chondrocalcinosis
Acromegaly
Hemachromatosis

Incongruity of Joint Surface/Malalignment
Slipped epiphysis
Congenital hip dislocation
Loose bodies
Genu valgum or varum
Aseptic necrosis

Neuropathic
Neurosyphilis
Leprosy

flares of symptoms are self-limited. It is not clear whether this is the natural course of the disease, whether the pain is caused by synovitis from hydroxyapatite crystals, or whether pain leads to resting of the joint and temporary resolution of symptoms. Pain from osteoarthritis, therefore, varies from day to day, but over years the course assumes a relatively constant slowly progressive contour that is quite distinct from the sine-wave variation of inflammatory diseases such as rheumatoid arthritis (Figure 1–1).

Joint enlargement resulting from osteophyte formation feels hard in comparison to the spongy feel of synovial proliferation. Deformity and subluxation result from bony overgrowth, loss of cartilage, and collapsed subchondral bone and cysts. Limitation of motion results from joint surface incongruity, muscle spasm, capsular contracture, and mechanical blockage from osteophytes or loose bodies.

Although most forms of osteoarthritis are not associated with inflammatory or systemic symptoms, generalized or erosive inflammatory osteoarthritis is recognized by many as a distinct clinical syndrome. It is characterized by signs of joint swelling, inflammation, and prolonged morning stiffness. It often involves multiple joints such as hands, knees, or hips, but need not be symmetrical. It responds well to antiinflammatory medications. It is sometimes difficult to differentiate this from rheumatoid arthritis or other causes of polyarthritis. Differentiating features that suggest inflammatory osteoarthritis include involvement of the distal interphalangeal joints, (which occurs in only 5% of patients with rheumatoid arthritis); lack of systemic symptoms such as fatigue, fever, and rash; and lack of anemia or positive rheumatoid factor. Synovial fluid should be examined to exclude polyarticular gout or pseudogout.

Osteoarthritis is such a ubiquitous process that the physician should always try to make another diagnosis or to look for biomechanical factors that can be corrected.

Although osteoarthritis is generally thought of as a noninflammatory arthropathy, occasional physical findings suggest inflammation, and the symptoms are improved with nonsteroidal antiinflammatory agents.

DIAGNOSTIC EVALUATION

The diagnosis of osteoarthritis is based on characteristic symptoms and x-ray evaluation of the weight-bearing joints and the spine. The four cardinal radiological features are: a) unequal loss of joint space, b) osteophytes, c) eburnation (juxtaarticular sclerosis), and d) subchondral bone cysts. However, the severity of pain in osteoarthritis correlates poorly with the radiological appearance of the joint. Features of osteoarthritis are common in x-rays, and, thus, another diagnosis should be considered if a) the complaint is not in a weight-bearing joint, or the carpometacarpal or distal interphalangeal joints; b) systemic symptoms exist; c) neuromotor or vascular symptoms are present; d) symptoms have been present for less than a month or are of acute onset; or e) there is synovitis. Physical findings are scarce in early osteoarthritis. In more advanced disease, boney enlargement and fixed deformities are the principal features.

Laboratory tests are normal in primary osteoarthritis and therefore are useful only when a diagnosis other than osteoarthritis is suggested by the clinical findings.

The approach to osteoarthritis varies according to the site of involvement.

Hand

Involvement of the hand is characterized by bony proliferation and the absence of objective synovitis in the small joints of the fingers: Heberden's nodes (in the distal interphalangeal joints) and Bouchard's nodes (in the proximal interphalangeal joints). Early symptoms usually include aching, discomfort, and stiffness, increased by heavy finger use. Metacarpophalangeal joints are rarely involved, except for the first carpometacarpal (the base of the thumb), which produces pain that is increased by forceful gripping and twisting movements of the hands. Carpometacarpal osteoarthritis is treated conservatively by splinting of the joint. X-ray evaluation of Heberden's and Bouchard's nodes is unnecessary.

Hip

Approximately 60% of patients with osteoarthritis of the hip complain of pain in the area of the greater trochanter and, less frequently, pain in the groin, back of the thigh, low back, or referred to the knee. The pain and stiffness associated with early osteoarthritis of the hip usually follow immobility and periods of excessive weight bearing.

The hip is relatively inaccessible to examination by observation or palpation. The earliest abnormality is reduced internal rotation (normal internal rotation is 35° to 45°), and abduction (normal is 45° to 50°). With progression of disease, hip motion is restricted in all directions, and the hip is flexed and foreshortened.

Important negative findings include absence of abnormality in other joints and a normal neuromuscular and vascular examination. Areas about the hip should be palpated for discrete tenderness secondary to bursitis, tendinitis, or muscle spasm. If the pain is reproduced by pressure over the greater trochanter, trochanteric bursitis is the cause of the pain.

Some believe that unequal leg length may cause osteoarthritis of the hip. A difference greater than 1 inch can cause hip pain by placing stress on the abductor muscles of the longer leg. Because the leg on the involved side is generally shortened by disease, the finding of a longer leg on the symptomatic side suggests that greater disparity existed before the onset of disease. Whether or not this theory is correct, a heel lift to about three quarters of the discrepancy is worth trying. This "rubber osteotomy" may relieve symptoms in about 15% of patients.

The earliest x-ray finding of osteoarthritis of the hip is unequal narrowing of the joint space. Minor narrowing may be detected if there is a difference in width of greater than 1 mm between the joint spaces of the normal and affected sides. If bilateral narrowing is present, unequivocal narrowing must be present before the diagnosis can be made with confidence. The joint space is probably abnormal if it is less than 4 mm in patients under age 70 or less than 3 mm in patients over 70. Osteophytes alone are not diagnostic of osteoarthritis, nor is there a relation between the presence of osteophytes and clinical symptoms. Primary osteoarthritis of the hip may be classified into two prognostic groups by the radiological picture: superolateral and medial. With superolateral disease, persistent unilateral involvement and progressive symptoms are the rule. In the medial form of osteoarthritis, involvement is usually bilateral initially or with time, and progression is variable.

Knee

Osteoarthritis of the medial and lateral compartments of the knee produces pain after weight bearing, particularly climbing and descending stairs, and rising from a sitting position. Patellofemoral osteoarthritis symptoms (Figure 3–2) are suggested when tensing the quadriceps, increasing the forces across the joint. Symptoms are therefore worse going down stairs than going up and worse rising from a chair than with level walking. Another symptom of patellofemoral osteoarthritis is night pain; patients push off against the bed when turning over, forcing the patella against the patellofemoral groove. The diagnosis of knee osteoarthritis is made by a) eliminating other possible causes of knee pain such as pes anserine or patellar bursitis, tendinitis, internal derangement, inflammatory joint disease, joint instability, and referred pain from hip disorders; and b) finding specific clinical and x-ray evidence of osteoarthritis. A weight-bearing film of both knees provides the most sensitive method of looking for cartilage loss in the medial and lateral compartments and of assessing the amount of varus or valgus deformity. Both anteroposterior and lateral views are necessary. Both knees should be included in the x-rays to evaluate the importance of radiological changes. Skyline views are necessary to evaluate the patellofemoral joint space.

Spine

Virtually everyone has pathological evidence of osteoarthritis of the spine by age 70, occurring in the vertebrae or posterior diarthrodial joints. The most commonly involved areas are the lower cervical spine (C6–C7) and the lower lumber spine (L3–L5, S1). Osteoarthritis of the spine produces poorly localized pain, which may radiate along the paraspinal areas and extend to the buttocks. Nerve-root encroachment by an osteophyte or irritation by synovitis may produce neurological symptoms. If the spinal cord is compressed or the spinal canal space is narrowed for any reason, upper motor neuron symptoms may develop (spinal stenosis). Stiffness and a decreased range of motion are common symptoms as well. On examination, stiffness, crepitus, local pain and tenderness, and muscle spasm may be present. In the neck, lateral flexion, rotation, and extension are usually more limited than forward flexion. Two very common syndromes occur in the cervical spine: compression of the sixth cervical nerve and compression of the seventh cervical nerve. In the former, one may note weakness in the biceps on shoulder flexion and in the wrist extensors by testing the wrist extension against resistance. There is diminished biceps deep-tendon reflex and diminished sensation to the thumb and index finger. In compression of the seventh cervical nerve, one notes weakness of the triceps by testing extension against resistance, a diminished triceps deep tendon reflex, and diminished sensation to the index and middle fingers.

In the lumbar spine, L4–L5 and L5–S1 are most commonly involved. Acute symptoms may be superimposed on chronic mechanical low back pain. Severe loss of spinal mobility usually does not occur until late in the disease.

Involvement of the spine by osteoarthritis requires anteroposterior and lateral and oblique x-ray views. Diagnostic findings include straightening or reversal of lordosis, narrowing of the intervertebral disc spaces with anterior and posterior osteophytes, laterally situated osteophytes on the vertebral bodies, deformity of the vertebral bodies, sclerosis, and encroachment on the intervertebral foramina by osteophytes and malaligned vertebral bodies. The oblique radiographs help in evaluation of facet joint osteoarthritis and are of little value in other situations.

TREATMENT STRATEGY

In the medical management of osteoarthritis, the natural history of the disease must be kept in mind. For example, osteoarthritis of the fingers does not lead to crippling or marked loss of function. Although osteoarthritis of the weight-bearing joints, especially in unilateral disease, is more likely to progress, one third of cases do not.

Preservation of function and reduction of pain are the major goals of management. The therapeutic plan should begin with an evaluation of the effect of the disease on the patient's life. What necessary activities can't the patient do? Does the pain interfere with work, play, or sleep, and how much discomfort is experienced with these activities? Treatable components of joint symptoms such as bursitis and tendinitis should be identified, and biomechanical factors, which may exacerbate the degenerative process, should be corrected.

Biomechanical Factors

Early treatment in osteoarthritis of the hip or knee should be directed at correction of biomechanical problems that accelerate the degenerative processes. If a discrepancy in leg length exists, a trial of therapy with a heel wedge of equivalent height may reduce symptoms considerably. Appliances such as canes and crutches are very helpful. For example, a static force of 385 pounds on one hip may be reduced to 66 pounds with a downward push on a cane of 38 pounds. Quadriceps-strengthening exercises in osteoarthritis of the knee are useful in providing additional support to the joint. Weight reduction should be recommended, although it is often difficult to achieve. In normal gait, three to five times the body weight is distributed across the knee or hip, and even a modest weight loss can reduce this force considerably.

Osteoarthritis of the cervical or lumbosacral spine may be painful because of nerve entrapment, muscle spasm, and/or joint inflammation. General measures include a cervical collar and cervical traction for cervical spine pain. For lumbosacral spine pain, useful general measures include instructions on techniques to reduce stresses on the back, isometric exercises for the abdominal muscles, and stretching of the hip flexors. A custom-made corset, is helpful, but should be used only for limited periods to prevent disuse atrophy of the muscles supporting the spine. In acute pain, muscle spasm, or nerve entrapment, the mainstays of treatment are bed rest and analgesics.

Local Measures

In general, cold is likely to be useful in acute musculoskeletal pain and heat in subacute pain. There is no proof that deep heat is better than superficial heat. There is no advantage of one type of superficial heat over another (moist heat, hot packs, hot soaks, paraffin, hot mud). Heating pads should be discouraged because patients may fall asleep during the application and suffer first-degree burns. Relative contraindications to heat include sensory neuropathies and circulatory impairment.

In patients with osteoarthritis of the hands, avoiding excessive finger use, such as in crocheting, is sometimes all that is required for symptomatic relief. Local symptomatic relief may be achieved by soaking the hands in warm water in the morning and using nylon spandex stretch gloves at night. Osteoarthritis of the first carpometacarpal joint responds well to thumb splinting. Rarely is suregery necessary, but persons with refractory pain may be considered for joint osteoplasty or arthrodesis. Neither is ideal and both require lengthy treatment. In patients with Heberden's and Bouchard's nodes, occasionally one joint is symptomatic out of proportion to the others, and local steroid injection into the joint or an overlying mucinous cyst may offer temporary benefit.

Steroid Injections

A careful search for pes anserine bursitis, trochanteric bursitis, or tendinitis is useful, because these conditions respond to local steroid injection. Intraarticular steroids usually have little role in osteoarthritis of the hip or knee, but can be tried if there is clinical evidence of synovitis (caused by intraarticular debris). Steroid injection of the hip is a difficult procedure and should be undertaken only by a skilled person. Steroid injections should not be done more than six times in the life of a joint and not within 6 weeks before joint surgery.

Drug Therapy

Early, mild osteoarthritis can be treated with analgesics alone, as can advanced disease where clinical sings of inflammation are not evident.

Antiinflammatory medication is useful in osteoarthritis with swelling, stiffness, and warmth. Aspirin and most nonsteroidal antiinflammatory drugs (NSAIDs) are comparable in their effects and can be used intermittently. Some evidence suggests that prolonged use of NSAIDs may accelerate cartilage degeneration. All the NSAIDs have similar side effects, which include gastrointestinal intolerance, fluid retention, platelet abnormalities, and hepatic and renal dysfunction (see Chapter 5). Both patient tolerance to side effects and individual therapeutic response may vary from one preparation to another. Therefore, one may be effective when others fail, and, if necessary, several alternatives should be tried. In general, NSAID changes should involve class switching (Table 5–3). For the majority of patients, flares are self-limited, and aggressive medication is rarely necessary. Patients should be educated to use aspirin and NSAIDs in a way that best enables them to function with their disease, but avoids the use of more than one drug at a time. Overlapping NSAIDs and salicylates increases the risk of serious gastrointestinal bleeding without increasing analgesia.

Surgery

When joint destruction is advanced and pain or disability is refractory to conservative treatment, total joint replacement should be considered (Table 6–2). An "end-stage" joint is likely when the patient is prevented from sleep or minimal weight bearing by pain, requires narcotics for pain, or has an unacceptable functional limitation. Other considerations include whether the damaged joint is the primary limiting condition, whether total joint replacement will outlive the patient, and whether there are other treatment options. In the young

TABLE 6–2. INDICATIONS FOR SURGERY IN OSTEOARTHRITIS

1. Refractory pain
2. Unacceptable disability
3. One single, worst joint that is rate limiting to patient
4. Bone-on-bone crepitus

patient with medial compartment narrowing and varus deformity of the knee, osteotomy may be recommended as a procedure to postpone total joint replacement. Contraindications to total joint replacement include youth (greater physical activity may hasten loosening, requiring revision surgery), lack of motivation (recovery after total joint replacement requires vigorous physical therapy), the presence of active infection or severe neurosensory deficits, and inadequate "bone stock" to properly seat the prosthesis.

Pain relief is achieved in more than 90% of patients who undergo total joint replacement of the knee and hip. Clinical failure requiring revision surgery occurs in approximately 2% of patients. Operative mortality ranges from 0.5% to 1.9%; facilities treating 50 patients per year or fewer have a higher mortality. Morbidity is less than 4%, and complications include pulmonary emboli, loosening of the prosthesis with time, deep or superficial infection, and dislocation.

For total joint replacement to be successful, patients must have a clear understanding of the goals. Physical activity is not completely normal after total joint replacement, and patients often must modify habits that place the prosthetic hip or knee at risk of dislocation. The best results in total joint replacement require careful patient selection, medical follow-up, patient education, and rehabilitation management.

REFERENCES

Altman R, Fries JF, Bloch DA et al.: Radiographic assessment of progression in OA. Arth Rheum 30:1214–1225, 1987.

Baron M, Dutil E, Berkson L, Lander P, Becker R: Hand function in the elderly: Relation to osteoarthritis. J Rheum 14:815–819, 1987.

Bland JH, Stulberg SD: Osteoarthritis: Pathology and clinical patterns. In WN Kelley et al. (eds), *Textbook of Rheumatology*. WB Saunders, Philadelphia, 1981, pp 1471–1490.

Felson DT, Naimark A, Anderson J, Kazis L, Castelli W, Meenan RF: The prevalence of knee osteoarthritis in the elderly: The Framingham osteoarthritis study. Arth Rheum 30:914–918, 1987.

Gofton JP: Studies in osteoarthritis of the hip. Part I. Classification. Can Med Assoc J 104:679–683, 791–799, 911–915, 1007–1011, 1971.

Liang MH, Cullen KE, Poss R: Primary total hip or knee replacement: Evaluation of patients. Ann Intern Med 97:735–739, 1982.

Moskowitz RW, Howell DS, Goldberg VM, Mankin HJ: *Osteoarthritis: Diagnosis and Management*. WB Saunders, Philadelphia, 1984.

Sheon RP, Moskowitz RW, Goldberg VM: Soft tissue rheumatic pain: Recognition, management, prevention. Lea & Febiger, Philadelphia, 1982, pp 172–202.

7

Diffuse Aches and Pains and Fibromyalgia/Fibrositis

The majority of patients who have diffuse aches and pains usually have a benign self-limited syndrome associated with various infectious diseases, primarily viral, or soft-tissue syndromes (Table 7–1).

To sort out such complaints, the history and physical usually suffice (Table 7–2), along with a limited laboratory evaluation (Table 7–3), particularly an erythrocyte sedimentation rate in the elderly patient. The history is directed towards identifying precipitating factors such as a prodromal illness, associated constitutional symptoms, or repetitive tasks. The examination is done to locate the anatomical site causing the symptoms and to differentiate intraarticular from extraarticular causes (Figure 1–2); and, if the pain is extraarticular, to determine whether the point of pain corresponds to a tendon or a bursa. Some symptoms in the history of a patient with diffuse aches and pains are red flags for systemic or metabolic diseases. Gelling or morning stiffness (particularly if longer than 30 minutes) is a symptom seen in inflammatory conditions such as polymyalgia rheumatica, rheumatoid arthritis (RA), systemic lupus erythmatosus (SLE), and some inflammatory muscle disease. Diffuse aches and pains without localizing physical findings may occur in these disorders and in the myopathies associated with endocrine disorders and metabolic bone disease (particularly osteomalacia).

An important and common systemic inflammatory disease is polymyalgia rheumatica (PMR) or giant cell arteritis with polymyalgia rheumatica. Polymyalgia rheumatica should always be considered in a patient over the age of 50 who develops aches and pains of the shoulder and hip girdle muscles. It is a myalgia without physical findings of muscle tenderness or weakness. Occasionally synovitis of small joints may be seen, which makes it difficult to differentiate it from an inflammatory polyarthritis. A frozen shoulder from painful myalgias may be seen. By definition, an elevated Westergren erythrocyte sedimentation rate greater than 50 mm/hr, and usually over 70 mm/hr, is part of the syndrome. A condition of unknown cause, the symptoms and the erythrocyte sedimentation rate

TABLE 7–1. DIFFERENTIAL DIAGNOSIS OF DIFFUSE ACHES/PAINS

Postviral arthralgias/myalgias
Bilateral soft-tissue rheumatism
Overuse syndromes
Fibrositis
Hypothyroidism
Metabolic bone disease
Paraneoplastic syndrome
Myopathy (polymyositis, dermatomyositis)
Rheumatoid arthritis, Sjogren's syndrome
Polymyalgia rheumatica with or without temporal arteritis
Hypermobility
Benign arthralgias/myalgias
Chronic fatigue syndrome
Hypophosphatemia

TABLE 7–2. DIFFUSE ACHES AND PAINS — RED FLAGS

Clinical Features	Significance
Age > 50	Polymyalgia rheumatica, paraneoplastic syndrome
Constitutional symptoms	Inflammatory disease Vasculitis, sepsis, malignancy
Weakness	Myopathy, endocrinopathy
Gelling	Inflammatory rheumatic disorder
New headache Claudication Visual symptoms Tender, nodular, thickened or reddened temporal artery	Temporal arteritis

TABLE 7–3. LABORATORY EVALUATION OF DIFFUSE ACHES AND PAINS

Complete blood count
Westergren erythrocyte sedimentation rate
Tetraiodothyronine or thyroid-stimulating hormone
Creatine phosphokinase or aldolase (if weakness)
Calcium, phosphate

are dramatically sensitive to low-dose steroids (i.e., prednisone under 20 mg/day); the symptoms usually improve within 24 to 48 hours, and the erythrocyte sedimentation rate improves within a week of starting steroids. To a less dramatic degree, nonsteroidal antiinflammtory drugs are effective in about a quarter of patients. Once an elevated erythrocyte sedimentation rate is identified in a patient with aches and pains, other systemic diseases need careful differentation. Chief among these are: early rheumatoid arthritis, systemic lupus erythematosus, polymyositis, paraneoplastic syndrome and giant-cell arteritis with polymyalgia rheumatica.

Polymyalgia rheumatica overlaps with giant-cell arteritis in about 10% to 40% of cases, but unless the patient has abnormalities of the temporal arteries or its branches such as redness, nodularity or pain, headache, visual disturbance, ischemia or claudication of the masseter muscles or tongue, or other organ system or systemic symptoms, the general recommendation is to *not* biopsy the temporal arteries. Careful examination of the temporal artery can be useful in targeting an artery for biopsy and for making a presumptive diagnosis of giant-cell arteritis. A reddened and tender artery occurs in less than 10% of cases of giant cell arteritis now seen. The findings of a potentially involved artery are the lack of a pulse, tenderness, nodularity, or a cord. Both branches and both sides should be palpated through their course as skip lesions occur. If the temporal artery can still be palpated after it is compressed against the temporalis fascia and/or the pulse obliterated, giant-cell arteritis or atherosclerosis are the two possibilities. If giant-cell arteritis is suspected, prednisone 1 mg/kg body weight in divided doses should be started and the biopsy obtained within several days. Blindness, the major morbidity, can occur with devastating rapidity. Once an eye is involved, the contralateral eye is also at considerable risk of becoming involved.

The treatment of polymalagia rheumatica, giant-cell arteritis or other inflammatory conditions should be done with someone experienced in their diagnosis. Experience is also needed for the tapering of steroids, since the long-term treatment has considerable toxicity. Generally, more attention is paid to following the erythrocyte sedimentation rate during the first 3 months of corticosteroids, and less attention is paid to fluctuations in erythrocyte sedimentation rate that occur later during the tapering phase. The duration of treatment averages 2 years.

Regardless of the etiologic diagnosis of generalized aching, the goal of the visit is to explain the pain, that is, to identify the anatomical sources of the pain. If one cannot either explain the pain anatomically or the pain does not go away, an expectant approach with follow-up is required. A variety of musculoskeletal symptoms can be the primary presenting symptom of people with malignancies or other systemic illnesses. Frequently at the outset, the cause may not be obvious, and it is only with follow-up and response to other clues that the diagnosis can eventually be made.

In general, symptoms and an examination that show *asymmetric* musculoskeletal pain are likely to lead to a diagnosis of internal derangement, tendinitis, or bursitis, i.e., a local problem, whereas a symmetrical presentation does not exclude the possibility of a regional cause but raises the possibility of a generalized systemic or metabolic disorder (Table 7–1).

FIBROSITIS/FIBROMYALGIA (Table 7–4)

When the patient has diffuse aches without a systemic, rheumatic, or endocrine illness, infection, local tendinitis, bursitis, or a ligamentous problem, fibrositis may be the diagnosis. The typical patient is healthy and complains of diffuse

TABLE 7–4. CLINICAL MANIFESTATIONS OF FIBROMYALGIA SYNDROME

Musculoskeletal Symptoms
Diffuse aches, pains, or stiffness
Weather sensitivity
Tender spots
Other Symptoms
Fatigue
Nonrestorative sleep
Irritable bowel symptoms
Muscle contraction headaches
Premenstrual syndrome
Anxiety/stress
Depression
Upper extremity numbness
Physical Examination
Tender points (usually four or more).
Cutaneous hyperemia at sites of tender-point palpation
Skin-roll tenderness (sometimes)

TABLE 7–5. TENDER POINTS

Upper fold of trapezius
Second costochondral junction
Epicondyles
Supraspinatus
Interspinous ligaments C4–C6
Interspinous ligaments L4–S1
Gluteus medius
Medial fat pad of knee

aches and pains that do not correspond to any specific anatomical site without objective findings, except for "tender points" (Figure 7–1 and Table 7–5), who has sleep disturbance but no other functional limitations and who has no laboratory abnormalities. These patients are a tremendous challenge to the specialist and generalist, and require the patience of Job to manage. Although no physical dysfunction is evident, many patients have a persistent course for many years.

The etiology of fibrositis is unknown. Some believe that fibrositis results in sleep disturbance rather than being the result. Deprivation of non-REM sleep in healthy individuals results in morning achiness, but treating the sleep disturbance may not always be successful. Clinical trials showed low-dose amitriptyline and cyclobenzaprine (10 to 30 mg/day) at bedtime improves the symptoms of fibrositis over the short term, but the longer benefit is not well maintained. A number of abnormalities of metabolism involving estrogens, endorphins, enkephalins, and urinary catecholamines have been invoked with scant evidence. Muscle biopsies done of tender points when compared to nontender points in

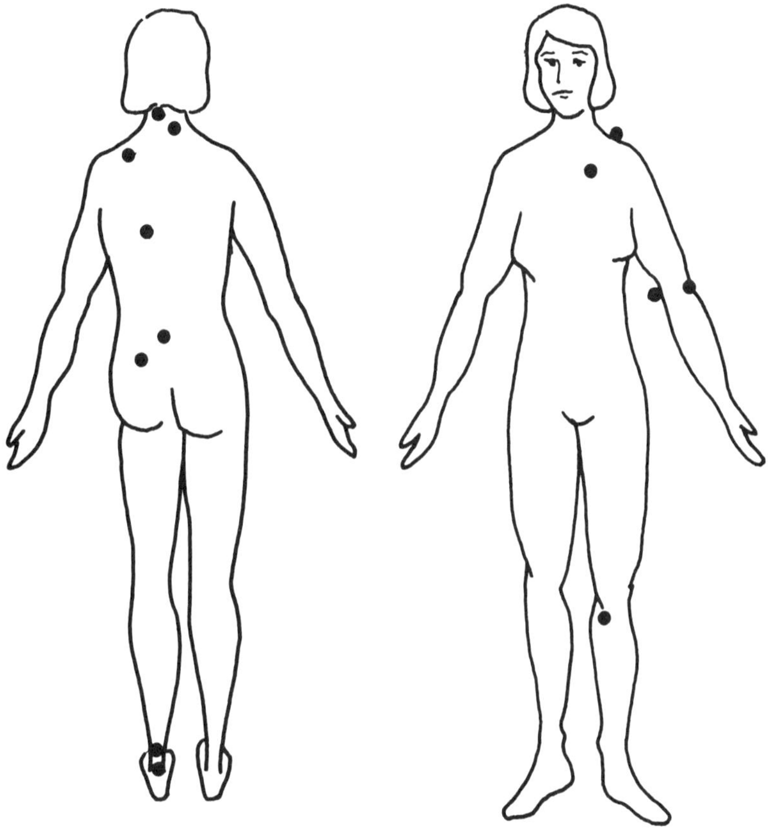

Figure 7–1. Fibrositis tender points. Points above the waist are found more frequently. Most patients with fibrositis have at least four such points.

the same patient or healthy controls show reduced high-energy phosphate compounds. A camp of experts believe that fibrositis results from trigger points and suggest local injection of these tender nodules with local anaesthetic agents and steroids. Many patients improve from trigger-point injection, but results are not predictable and are frequently short lived. Randomized trials have shown that saline injection is at least as good as steroid injection of trigger points. Aerobic training seems to help some patients. Amitriptyline, cyclobenzaprine and aerobic training are the only three therapies shown to have benefit in randomized controlled trials. Corticosteroids and NSAIDs are of no apparent benefit, although NSAIDs may provide analgesia. As with many unexplained disorders, psychosomatic factors have been thought to be important in pathogenesis, but many well-adjusted individuals with no secondary gain have disabling prolonged fibrositis. A variety of immunological abnormalities, such as immune complexes, autoantibodies, etc., have been found in some patients with fibrositis, but these findings are not reproducible and do not exist in all patients.

Patients who are anxious or fear serious illness should be managed with reassurance and patient education. Many times the issue for these patients are not fear of dreaded illness, but frustration with physicians who do not acknowledge their pain or who have attributed it to psychological problems. The therapy here, then, is attentive listening and acknowledgment of the patient's symptoms. The label, *fibrositis*, provides legitimacy and counters anxiety over the perceived possibility of a life-threatening disorder.

To provide reassurance, one needs to explain fibrositis, explain what to expect, and outline a treatment strategy. It is also useful to emphazise to the patient's what they do *not* have. Asking patient's what their fears are, or what they think the diagnosis is, may uncover these and may facilitate a discussion to deal with these fears.

Allaying fears and anxieties can only be done with a calm, firm, and definitive approach. If the patient is confident in the physician and can sense the physician's confidence in the diagnosis, and understands what to expect and the plan of the treatment, much can be done to improve the mental outlook.

Aerobic exercise should be recommended and physical modalities emphasizing stretching and massage are useful. Having stretching and massage without the conditioning program rarely work. Patients with sleep disturbance can be treated with sleep medications or preferably tricyclic antidepressants such as amitriptyline (25–50 mg). Some patients with fibrositis can be exquisitely sensitive to doses that would not normally be expected to be therapeutic, such as 12.5 mg of amytriptyline. Nonsteroidals rarely seem to help.

REFERENCES

Ahles TA, Ynus MB, Riley SD, Bradley JM, Masi AT. Psychological factors associated with primary fibromyalgia syndrome. Arthritis Rheum 27:1101–1106, 1984.

Campbell SM, Clark S, Tindall EA, Forehand ME, Bennett RM: Clinical characteristics of fibrositis. Arthritis Rheum 26:817–824, 1983.

Carette S, McCain GA, Bell DA, Fam AG: Evaluation of amitriptyline in primary fibrositis. Arth-ritis Rheum 29:655–659, 1986.

Frost FA, Jessen B, Siggaard–Anderson J: A control, double-blind comparison of mepivacaine injection versus saline injection for myofascial pain. Lancet 1:499–500, 1980.

Goldenberg DL: Fibromyalgia syndrome. An emerging but controversial conditon. JAMA 257:2782–2787, 1987.

Goldenberg DL, Dinerman H, Felson D: A randomized clinical trial of naproxen and amitriptyline in the treatment of patients with fibromyalgia. Arthritis Rheum 29:1371–1377, 1986.

Healey LA, Wilse KR: *The Systemic Manifestations of Temporal Arteritis.* Grune Stratton, New York, 1987.

Robb–Nicholson C, Chang RW, Anderson S, Roberts WN, Longine J, Corson J, Larson M, George D, Green J, Bryant G, Liang MH: Diagnostie value of the history and physical examination in giant cell arteritis. A clinical pathological study of 81 temporal artery biopsies. J Rheum 15:1793–1796, 188.

In McCarty DJ (ed). *Arthritis and allied condition* 10th edition. Lea and Febiger, Philadelphia, 1985, p 1083.

Travell J: Myofascial pain and dysfunction. In Travell JG, Simons DG (eds). *Myofascial Pain and dysfunction: The Trigger Point Manual.* Williams & Wilkins, Baltimore, 1983 pp 1901.

Wilke WS, Mackenzie AH: Proposed pathogenesis of fibrositis. Cleveland Clin Quart 52:147–154, 1985.

Wysenbeck AJ, Mor F, Lurie Y, Weinberg A: Imipramine for the treatment of fibrositis: A therapeutic trial. Ann Rheum Dise 44:752–753, 1985.

8

Gout and Other Crystalline Arthropathies

Crystal-induced arthropathies is a group of diseases caused by the inflammatory properties of various crystals. Characteristics held in common by gout (caused by monosodium urate crystals), pseudogout (calcium pyrophosphate crystals), and hydroxyapatite crystal disease are their clinical presentation as acute monoarticular arthritis or oligoarthritis. Their diagnosis is by the demonstration of the crystals in the joint fluid. All respond to nonsteroidal antiinflammatory agents and steroids. Gout responds dramatically and almost specifically to colchicine. The biology of gout has been exquisitely elucidated. There is considerable controversy, as yet unresolved, as to whether calcium pyrophosphate and hydroxyapatite are the primary cause of inflammatory arthritis or the result of aging, previous cartilage damage, or mild preexisting inflammatory disease.

In any case, the understanding of crystalline synovitidies, particulary gout, represents an important advance in modern rheumatology and management is highly effective.

EPIDEMIOLOGY

Gout is generally a disease of middle-aged or older men and postmenopausal women, particularly women on thiazide diuretics. Its incidence follows an increasing incidence of mild elevation of serum uric acid in older people. Most patients with gout have an onset of their disease after the age of 40. Patients with a younger onset may have inherited disorders of metabolism associated with hyperuricemia. Acute attacks of gout tend to be more frequent with increasing age if they are not treated.

Calcium pyrophosphate deposition occurs in a large number of elderly people without symptoms. About 5% of people who are of retirement age will have linear deposits of their fibrocartilage on x-ray, and this percentage rises to a quarter of the population in people who are 90 or older.

Hydroxyapatite disease often occurs in people who have high calciumphoshate serum calcium and phosphate products, and therefore is most common in people with renal failure. It has also been identified in some cases of "acute" osteoarthritis and in persons with acute bursitis of the shoulder when it is looked for.

DIAGNOSIS OF GOUT

The diagnosis of gout should be considered in patients with monoarticular arthritis, especially involving the first MTP joint (podagra) and other joints of the feet. Polyarthritis is an uncommon presentation of gout and is usually asymmetric. In women, polyarticular gout is frequently associated with thiazide-induced hyperuricemia. Gouty inflammation can be confused with cellulitis because of the marked erythema and swelling, but gouty pain, unlike cellulitis, prevents sleep and occurs at rest. A history of a uric acid stone or gout in other members of the family and hyperuricemia increase the likelihood of gout, but, ultimately, the diagnosis must be made by the demonstration of monosodium urate crystals in the joint fluid.

Hyperuricemia is not gout. Hyperuricemia is a necessary but not sufficient condition for the diagnosis of gout. Although hyperuricemia increases the risk of gout, most individuals with hyperuricemia will never have gout and urate deposition in their tissues. They have asymptomatic hyperuricemia and need not be treated.

Only a single drop of joint fluid is necessary for the identification of the diagnostic crystals, which appear as needle-shaped 2 to 10-micron long crystals. Large numbers of crystals are generally present in the fluid during an acute attack, and they have also been demonstrated in individuals between gouty flares. The crystals are strongly birefringent and display negative birefringence when viewed with a compensated polarized-light microscope and a first-order red compensator. (See p 93.) Sharply defined erosions of subchondral bone with a bony shelf above on radiographic examination is also helpful in distinguishing gout from other forms of chronic arthritis.

The severity and rate of progression of untreated gout are extremely variable. Some individuals have no more than a few attacks in a lifetime, and others have recurrent attacks with few asymptomatic intervals, erosive disease, and multiple joints involved, along with deposits of monosodium urate in the soft tissues (tophaceous deposits).

MANAGEMENT

The management of a patient requires that the acute attack be controlled and that a long-term strategy be devised. The maintenance of a normal uric acid in most patients requires lifelong treatment, and it is important that the patient and physician understand the rationale for treating this disease and commit themselves to monitoring the treatment.

The acute gouty episode can be managed with a host of agents, including oral and intravenous colchicine, a variety of nonsteroidal antiinflammatory agents, and corticosteroids. Colchicine is an inexpensive and highly effective agent. Its effect on gout is so predictable that its effectiveness can be used to support the diagnosis of gout. Colchicine is a dangerous drug when used casually. Patients who are older or who have renal and hepatic insufficiency should be given much smaller doses. Colchicine is bound to body tissues and someone who is on oral colchicine must have a much smaller dose of either oral or intravenous colchicine during an acute attack.

For the patient with a fully developed acute attack, 0.6 mg of colchicine can be given every hour until the patient has relief or develops side effects such as nausea or diarrhea. No more than 12 tablets should be given for any single acute attack in a 24-hour period, and the total dose should be lowered for individuals with renal and hepatic disease. The best responses to colchicine occur when it is given early. Colchicine may also be administered intravenously but its use in the office is not necessary and is not recommended.

Nonsteroidal antiinflammatory drugs are at least as effective as colchicine for the relief of acute gouty arthritis. Indomethocin, ibuprofen, fenoprofen, naprosyn, tolmetin, sulindac, and piroxicam have all been shown to be effective in the management of acute gouty arthritis. The maximum recommended dose should be used as early as possible during an acute attack, and when the symptoms have subsided the drug should be gradually tapered.

For severe persistent attacks, corticosteroids may be required. Oral and injectable corticosteroids are particlarly useful adjuncts in patients with renal insufficiency. Every other drug used in acute or chronic gout — NSAIDs, allopurinol, colchicine — requires careful dose adjustment when employed in the presence of renal disease. Appreximately a third of patients treated with steroids have a flare of the disease after the therapy is stopped, and thus either a nonsteroidal antiinflammatory agent or colchicine should be used as prophylaxis to cover the steroid withdrawal. The usual prophylactic dose of colchicine is 0.6 mg twice daily, and for a nonsteroidal antiinflammatory agent it is usually half of the standard daily dose.

In the patient with recurrent attacks, and in patients with tophaceous deposits with hyperuricemia, there are two ways to lower serum urate concentration. One is uricosuric therapy and the other is using a xanthine oxidase inhibitor to reduce uric acid production. The object of uricosuric therapy is to increase the renal excretion of uric acid by blocking tubular resorption of urate, thereby reducing the serum urate concentration. To avoid the sudden exposure of the kidney to large quantities of uric acid and to prevent precipitation of an acute gout attack, the dose of the drug should be gradually increased over 7 to 10 days in the presence of alkalinized urine. Bicarbonate or Scholl's solution can be used to increase the urine pH.

Probenecid is the most widely used uricosuric agent and a 1 g daily dose results in a mean increase of 50% in the renal excretion of uric acid and a fall of a third of the serum urate concentration. The maximum recommended daily dosage is 3 g.

If toxicity occurs with probenecid, sulfinpyrazone can be used as a substitute. Both probenecid and sulfinpyrazone are generally well tolerated. The most common adverse reactions are gastric intolerance. One should note that administration of salicylates in any dosage neutralizes the uricosuric effect of both these agents.

Allopurinol, a xanthine oxidase inhibitor, as a single dose of 300 to 800 mg per day, promptly lowers serum uric acid within several days. Doses of allopurinal as low as 100 mg every third day are used for patients with renal failure. It is not a benign drug and can cause liver toxicity, interstitial nephritis, fever, rash, and transient leukopenia. An acute gout attack may be precipitated during the early stages of allopurinol therapy. This may be prevented with small doses of allopurinol, by gradually increasing the dose, or giving a prophylactic agent at the same time. The latter is probably the most widely used strategy.

The primary indications for allopurinol in patients with hyperuricemia and gout are:

1. Patients with uric acid kidney stones or excrete over 1000 mg of urate in 24 hours.
2. Patients with tophaceous gout who require both uricosuric agents and xanthine oxidase inhibition
3. Patients who respond poorly to uricosuric therapy or who cannot tolerate the uricosuric drug
4. Patients with hyperuricemia secondary to myeloproliferative disorders before induction therapy with cytotoxic drugs. Allopurinol prevents acute gouty nephropathy and renal insufficiency.

The treatment of patients between gout attacks may be observation alone or use of a low dose of colchicine (0.6 mg twice daily) or NSAID to prevent recurrences. A purine-free diet (essentially avoiding internal organs of animals) is not a very effective way of lowering serum uric acid. Medications and clinical states known to produce hyperuricemia should be avoided if possible in patients with gout. These include thiazides, low-dose salicylates, alcohol, or fasting.

Asymptomatic hyperuricemia is increasingly diagnosed since the wide use of multiphasic testing systems. There is no data that shows that untreated patients with asymptomatic hyperuricemia suffer any long-term consequences other than an increased risk of gout. Since acute gout is so well managed, there is little reason to treat asymptomatic hyperuricemia for this possibilty. In patients with a history of recurrent renal calculi with hyperuricemia, a 24-hour urine urid acid is indicated to determine if they are hyperexcretors of uric acid (i.e., urine uric acid 1000 mg/24 hours). Patients with hyperexcretion are at increased risk for developing uric acid renal calculi and should be treated with allopurinol and *not* with a uricosuric agent, which may cause acute precipitation of urate stones.

REFERENCES

Agudelo CA, Weinberger A, Schumacher HR, et al.: Definitive diagnosis of gout by identification of urate crystals in asymptomatic metatarsophalangeal joints. Arthritis Rheum 22:559–569, 1979.

Boss BG, Seegmiller JE: Hyperuricemia and gout: Classification, complications and management. N Engl J Med 300:1459–1468, 1976.

Liang MH, Fries JF: Asymptomatic hyperuricemia: The case for conservative management. Ann Intern Med 136:893–896, 1976.

Rakic MT, Valkenburg HA, Davidson RT, Engles JP, Miikkelsen WM, Neel JV, Duff IF, Himes S: Observations on the natural history of hyperuricemia and gout. I. An 18 year follow-up of 19 gouty families. Am J Med 37:862–871, 1964.

Roberts WN, Liang MH, Stern SH: Colchicine for acute gout: Assessment of risks and benefits. JAMA 257:1920–1922, 1987.

Wyngaarden JB, Kelley WN: *Gout and Hyperuricemia*. Grune & Stratton, New York, 1976.

9 Infectious Arthritis

Infections may cause joint symptoms by at least three mechanisms. Microorganisms can invade the joint space by the circulation or by contiguous spread, trigger an immunological process leading to arthritis after the evidence of infection is gone (acute rheumatic fever, Reiter's disease), or persist within a joint as nonviable components.

Infectious agents causing arthritis may be bacteria, virus, fungi, or mycobacteria and, to the degree that these infections can be specifically treated with antibiotics, are extremely important to recognize. Bacteria and fungi can destroy a joint as a result of local cellular responses to infections in which proteolytic enzymes are released. Some infections may induce synovitis long after the microorganism is eradicated.

Although spontaneous infections of the joint may occur, a variety of clinical settings are associated with an increased risk of joint sepsis. These include:

- arthritis
- prior joint surgery
- immunocompromised host
- bacteremia (pyelonephritis, bacterial endocarditis)

Signs of infection such as leukocytosis, elevated erythrocyte sedimentation rate, and fever may not be present, and the only way to make the diagnosis is to culture the joint fluid. Therefore, a joint aspiration is always required whenever there is a possibility of infectious arthritis. The fluid should be cultured in the appropriate medium and a gram stain should be done on fresh fluid. In suspected gonococcal arthritis, the synovial fluid should be plated on Thayer–Martin blood agar and put immediately under CO_2 to increase the yield of growth. The yield of cultures or gram stains depends on the specific infectious agent. For example, gonorrhoea is recovered in less than 50% of suspected individuals. Mycobacteria and fungi can be recovered in well over half of the patients simply by synovial fluid culture, but the diagnostic yield can be increased considerably by doing a synovial biopsy with culture and histology. Blood cultures should always be obtained because many infections of the joint are metastatic infections from other sources.

The optimal treatment of joint infections includes appropriate antibiotics, drainage, and joint rest. Identification of the organism is the key to successful treatment. Infections in closed spaces need to be drained. Closed-needle joint aspiration will suffice, except in hips and shoulders, where open drainage is usually required. All suspected or proven joint infections require consultation and hospitalization.

Early on, the joint should be immobilized with splints to help make the patient more comfortable, but exercises should be started as soon as pain subsides to prevent muscle atrophy and contractures. If the effusion is not resolving, joint aspiration should be repeated to reduce the volume of fluid, which prevents full extension of a joint.

Based on the rapidity of reaccumulation of the fluid, this regimen can vary from three arthrocenteses a day to one every 3 days. Evidence clearly shows that delay in drainage, particularly delay beyond 72 hours from the onset of symptoms, is the largest determinant of short-term outcome, i.e., whether the patient becomes septicemic and whether there are complications such as osteomyelitis and significant cartilage loss. A joint infection by *Staphylococcus aureus* can destroy cartilage in 48 hours. On the other end of the spectrum, most cases of gonococcal arthritis do not result in joint damage.

A falling joint-fluid cell count and minimal reaccumulation of fluid are indicative of a good clinical response. Repeated closed arthrocentesis with a needle can produce good results 80% of the time, but one should go to open drainage after 3 days if the patient is not substantially improved and if the volume of arthrosentesis fluid and the cell count in the fluid is not dropping rapidly.

Open drainage should be done early in certain situations. Infections in the hand are dangerous because compartment syndromes may develop rapidly. The shoulder has multiple anatomical compartments and may not be drained completely through a needle. Hips and shoulders always require surgical drainage.

Cellulitis overlying a joint may be difficult to differentiate from a septic joint. Pain from septic arthritis is due to stretching of the joint capsule and is equally painful in all ranges of motion. Whereas pain from cellulitis hurts most when the joint motion stretches the cellulitic area. Swelling and erythema in a septic joint occurs over the entire circumference of the joint line whereas cellutitis is more localized. When in doubt the joint should be tapped, since the patient will be on antibiotics anyway and the penalty for not treating a septic joint early is high.

Another question that commonly arises in the treatment of septic joints is the duration of antibiotic treatment. As a rule, gonococcal joint infections can be treated for 2 weeks, and all others are treated for a minimum of 4 to 6 weeks. Intraarticular antibiotics are not used because they create chemical inflammation and because the drug levels obtained by intravenous antibiotics are adequate.

Ancillary treatments are useful. Nonsteroidal antiinflammatory agents and joint rest help relieve pain. A continuous passive motion machine for a septic knee is useful to maintain the range of motion.

COMMON TYPES OF INFECTIOUS ARTHRITIS

Nongonococcal arthritis is caused by a variety of agents, chiefly *Staphylococcus aureus*, streptococcal species, and gram-negative bacilli. In children, hemophilus influenza is common.

Nongonococcal arthritis generally affects a single joint, most commonly a weight-bearing joint, and especially the knee. Most patients experience a rapid onset of arthritis, which, unlike most forms of inflammatory arthritis, is painful with range of motion in any direction. X-rays of the joint early on show only soft-tissue swelling. It may take weeks before other x-ray signs of periosteal elevation, bone destruction, and joint-space narrowing are seen. Gallium and bone scanning detect changes earlier than plain radiographs. Nuclear magnetic resonance imaging may be even more sensitive.

Patients with such infections tend to be very young or very old, and frequently are compromised hosts. In a patient with a polyarthritis, such an infection may be difficult to diagnose because it occurs on the background of multiple joint symptoms. When there is one joint that is painful out of proportion to the others and with local signs of inflammation unlike the others (particularly redness), one should suspect infection.

Gonococcal arthritis should be suspected in any person who is sexually active. The typical patient with gonococcal arthritis is a woman who presents around the time of the menses or pregnancy with migratory polyarthralgias and, very commonly, severe tenosynovitis, particularly of the wrists. A characteristic skin rash may occur in two–thirds of the patients and tends to be a scantily distributed painless macularpapular, pustular, vesicular, or bullous eruption, classically a gun-metal grey lesion on an erythematous bases it requires a careful search. Patients may have fever and signs of bacteremia during the early part of the disease but not always. As mentioned above, the organism can be recovered in less than half of the cases. Cervical, anal, oral, and blood cultures for gonococcus increase the yield but some cases are never confirmed. These are diagnosed by their prompt response to antibiotics.

Gonococcal arthritis may need to be separated from Reiter's syndrome in men. A typical hemorrhagic skin rash would favor gonococcus. Additional differential points include a preponderence of lower extremity involvement among patients with Reiter's syndrome. Gonococcal arthritis more commonly affects the upper extremity. Achilles' tendinitis, plantar faciitis, and uveitis are almost never seen in gonococcal arthritis but occur in Reiter's syndrome. Keratoderma blennorrhagica clinches the diagnosis of Reiter's syndrome. Gonococcal infection of the pharynx or rectum would favor a gonococcal arthritis, as would a true migratory pattern of presentation.

The question of whether the person with gonoccocal arthritis should be admitted to the hospital is made on the basis of social factors and whether the joint aspiration shows frankly purulent fluid. Patients with frankly purulant effusions, as opposed to synovitis with scant fluid; patients with diabetes; those with poor comprehension and with poor social supports; or those who do not have transportation or a phone should be admitted.

Effective antibiotic regimens for disseminated gonococcal infection (arthritis-dermatitis syndrome) include: procaine penicillin G, two million units IV every 4 hours until improvement plus ampicillin 500 mg orally four times a day for a total of 7 days of treatment; or ampicillin 3.5 g orally with 1 g of probenecid initially plus ampicillin 500 mg orally four times a day for a total of 1 week. The advantage of the third-generation cephalosporins is that they are effective against penicillin-resistant gonococci. For penicillin-allergic patients, tetracycline, erythromycin, and spectinomycin can be used. Tetracyclines should be avoided in pregnant patients. Tetracycline and related antibiotics are inadequate against anorectal gonococcal infections. Appropriate antibiotics usually reverse the symptoms within 24 to 48 hours. Repeated joint drainage of the effusion is seldom required.

Bacterial endocarditis may be associated with a septic arthritis, which is rare, or with a sterile, moderately severe inflammatory synovitis. The latter manifestation is probably due to hypersensitivity or an immune-mediated process. Polyarthritis and polyarthralgias, monoarthritis, myalgias, hypertrophic osteoarthropathy, disc infections, and low back pain are the musculoskeletal syndromes seen.

Tuberculous arthritis has declined in incidence but still occurs in immunocompromised patients, AIDS patients, alcoholics, and the growing number of homeless. Joint and bone infections occur from hematogenous spread and contiguous infection from infected bone. Classically, tuberculous arthritis presents as a chronic insidious monoarthritis with few of the typical findings of inflammation (a "cold abscess"). The most commonly involved sites are the vertebral column (Pott's disease) and weight-bearing joints. Chronic tenosynovitis may also be caused by mycobacteria species.

Treatment of tuberculous arthritis requires long-term administration of multiple antibiotics and should always be done with consultation. Fungal arthritis is also rare and has a clinical presentation similar to that of mycobacterial. Fungal infections of bone and joint include coccidioidomycosis, sporotrichosis, blastomycosis, and candidiasis.

Many viral arthritides have been described, including hepatitis B, parvovirus, rubella, and mumps. In general, viral arthritides result from hypersensitivity or immune complex disease. Clinically they look like rheumatoid arthritis and have tantalized investigators to link viruses and rheumatoid arthritis. Most of these arthritis syndromes resolve. Some viruses such as rubella and parvovirus may cause chronic synovitis in a small percentage of patients.

Lyme Disease

Lyme disease deserves comment as it is the most well-studied and most recently described arthritis associated, a spirochetal infection by *Borrielia burgdorferi*. It is clinically recognized by a characteristic skin lesion called erythema chronicum migrans (ECM), a red macularpapular rash that expands over time to form an annular lesion, which appears within 3 days to 3 weeks after an *Ixodes dammini* tick bite carrying the spirochete. ECM is often accompanied by chills, fever, malaise, fatigue, and headache or stiff neck. Weeks to months later, neurological, cardiac, and joint complications may occur. The histology of the lesions suggests that this is also an immune complex disorder. Joint symptoms occur in about 50% of patients bitten and include migratory polyarthritis without morning stiffness and tendonitis, and they may recur. Chronic monoarticular involvement of a large joint is less common.

Neurological abnormalities may occur within a few weeks after ECM, last for months, and usually resolve. These include aseptic meningitis or meningoencephalitis, chorea, cerebellar ataxia, cranial neuritis including bilateral Bell's palsy, motor and sensory neuropathy, radicular neuritis, and mononeuritis multiplex. Cardiac abnormalities also arise within a few weeks after ECM and include atrioventricular block and myopericarditis.

Penicillin G, tetracycline, doxycline, and ceftriaxone may prevent or attenuate subsequent arthritis. It is not yet clear that neurological, cardiac, or joint disease will respond to antibiotics.

REFERENCES

Espinoza L, Goldenberg DL, Arnett F, Alarcon G (eds): *Infections in the Rheumatic Diseases: A Comprehensive Review of Microbial Relations to Rheumatic Disorders.* Grune and Stratton, Orlando, FL, 1988.

Goldenberg DL, Reed JI: Bacterial arthritis. N Eng J Med 312:764–769, 1985.

Hyer FH, Gottlieb NC: Rheumatic disorders associated with viral infection. Semin Arthritis Rheum 8:17–31, 1978.

Brogadir SP, Schimmer BM, Myers AR: Spectrum of the gonococcal arthritis-dermatitis syndrome. Semin Arthritis Rheum 8:177–183, 1979.

Masi AT, Eisenstein BI: Disseminated gonococcal infection and gonococcal arthritis: II. Clinical manifestations, diagnosis, complications, treatment, and prevention. Semin Arthritis Rheum 10:173–197, 1981.

Steere AC, Schoen RT, Taylor E: The clinical evolution of Lyme arthritis. Ann Intern Med 107:725–731, 1987.

10

Rheumatoid Arthritis

Rheumatoid arthritis is a chronic systemic inflammatory illness and polyarthritis. It typically affects small joints in a symmetrical and additive pattern. It is an illness that may have extraarticular and systemic features of varying frequency and severity. The extraarticular manifestations include rheumatoid nodules, vasculitis, neuropathy, scleritis, lung involvement, lymphadenopathy, pericarditis, and splenomegaly.

Rheumatoid arthritis affects women two to three times as often as men and increases in prevalence with age up until the seventh decade. One to three percent of the population have rheumatoid arthritis.

CLINICAL PRESENTATIONS AND COURSE

Rheumatoid arthritis presents in varied ways, and its course ranges from mild illness involving only a few joints and of brief duration to a relentless, progressive, destructive polyarthritis with systemic vasculitis. At the outset, no pattern of joint or laboratory findings is completely reliable in predicting the course. However, poor function, destructive arthritis, and vasculitic complications are more frequent in patients with sustained high titres of rheumatoid factor, rheumatoid nodules, positive antinuclear antibody at any time in the course, uncontrolled synovitis, and hand-foot joint involvement. At the onset, rheumatoid arthritis may present with systemic symptoms such as fatigue, fever, anorexia, and weight loss, and the joint symptoms only manifest themselves later in the course. About 20% of patients have acute polyarthritis and systemic symptoms as their first manifestation of rheumatoid arthritis. Articular involvement in rheumatoid arthritis is manifested by pain and swelling. Patients with active rheumatoid arthritis complain of morning joint stiffness that generally lasts longer than 30 minutes, but some may have stiffness throughout the day.

Joint involvement in rheumatoid arthritis is generally symmetrical, although it may not be absolutely so at any given point. The most commonly involved joints in rheumatoid arthritis are the small joints of the hand, particularly the metacarpal and proximal interphalangeal joints, and the wrists, knees, and feet. A small percentage of patients with rheumatoid arthritis have pauciarticular or monoarticular disease (which usually involves the knees) for months to years. Any joint with synovium can be involved, including temporomondibular joints, elbows, shoulders, sternoclavicular joints, hips, ankles, subtalar joints, and the cervical spine. Back pain, a common complaint, is usually not due to rheumatoid arthritis.

Several patterns of disease activity are noted: an intermittent course, a long remission course, and a progressively destructive course. The intermittent course is marked by partial to complete remissions and is generally a mild disease. Another group undergoes a long clinical remission after therapy for rheumatoid arthritis and may have smouldering signs of inflammation, but have little destructive disease. The third group of patients has progressive destruction of multiple joints with disability with or without extraarticular manifestations. The latter group may be the most common.

It is the picture of progressive, crippling disease that patients fear when they hear their diagnosis. Therefore, it is important to address these concerns early, even if the patient does not raise these concerns spontaneously.

DIAGNOSIS

The diagnosis of rheumatoid arthritis is made on the basis of the history of swelling, stiffness, gelling, or pain in the small joints of the hand, which is persistent over 6 weeks and may be associated with systemic symptoms such as fatigue, anorexia, and weight loss. The physical exam of actively involved joints shows swelling, warmth, and some pain with range of motion. Early on in the disease, there may be limitation of motion from an increased volume of synovial fluid or pain. Classic findings of rheumatoid arthritis, such as ulnar deviation, swan neck, boutonniere deformity, and rheumatoid nodules take months or years to develop.

Extraarticular manifestations, such as scleritis or vasculitis, whether they occur either early or late in the disease, constitute a reason to refer the patient to a rheumatologist. (See the list of extraarticular manifestations in Table 10–1.)

The laboratory is not helpful in making the diagnosis of rheumatoid arthritis, particularly in the acute setting. The rheumatoid factor, if it is positive, may be helpful, but the number of false-positive rheumatoid factors increases with age, and between 10% and 20% of patients with clinical rheumatoid arthritis are consistently rheumatoid factor negative. The sedimentation rate is nonspecific and is helpful only for following therapy when the clinical signs are ambiguous. Synovial fluid is consistently inflammatory, but is not diagnostic. X-rays are not helpful in early disease but are very useful to assess structural damage. Six months of active synovitis are usually required before x-ray findings of erosions are manifested.

TABLE 10–1. EXTRAARTICULAR MANIFESTATIONS OF RHEUMATOID ARTHRITIS

Skin
Vasculitis
Rheumatoid nodules

Ophthalmic
Episcleritis
Scleritis
Scleromalacia perforans
Sicca syndrome

Pulmonary
Interstitial pneumonitis
Fibrosis
Pleuritis
Rheumatoid nodule

Cardiac
Myocarditis
Pericarditis
Coronary arteritis and aortitis
Valvulitis

Hematologic
Felty syndrome (rheumatoid arthritis, splenomegaly, leucopenia)
Lymphadenopathy
Anemia
Hyperviscosity

Neurologic
Peripheral neuropathy (including entrapment neuropathy)

Miscellaneous
Amyloidosis

THERAPY

Patient education is important. Patients fear loss of function or chronicity and require support. Their malady may not be obvious to family members, and it is important to talk to the family to achieve an understanding of what special problems the illness presents. The family should be reassured that most patients with rheumatoid arthritis have a productive life. With good care many options exist for control (not necessarily cure) of the disease. Patients need to gain mastery of their condition by learning how to monitor their disease, their medications, and function, and should be encouraged to be active within the limits of their capacities. Once the diagnosis has been made, referral to a rheumatologist may be helpful. A referral should always be made if gold, penicillamine, methotrexate or other disease-modifying therapy is contemplated or if steroids are

TABLE 10–2. REFERRAL CRITERIA FOR PATIENTS WITH RHEUMATOID ARTHRITIS

Loss of function
Refractory synovitis
Corticosteroid considered
Slow-acting disease-modifying agent (gold, methotrexate, penicillamine, azathioprine) considered
Rheumatoid vasculitis
Extraarticular manifestations

* See Table 1–1.

contemplated, the patient is deteriorating, or extraarticular manifestations are present (Table 10–2).

In assessing function, find out what patients expect to be able to do and what their career, family, and recreational needs are (Table 1–1). In assessing a patient's overall well-being, pay attention to fatigue, the amount of morning stiffness, appetite, weight loss, etc. These nonspecific symptoms may herald a flare or reflect disease activity.

A stepped approach to the pharmacological management of rheumatoid arthritis is based on a program of psychosocial support, appropriate resting of active joints, and physical and occupational therapy. Antiinflammatory doses of salicylates or nonsteroidal antiinflammatory agents are pushed to efficacy or toxicity. Failing this or for severe cases, disease-modifying antirheumatic drugs (DMARDs) should be considered. These include oral gold, parenteral gold, penicillamine, cyclophosamide, methotrexate, and azathioprine. Steroids should be used in select situations and in the lowest dose possible. Some side effects of these medications need comment. Tinnitus or impaired hearing occurs above the therapeutic range of salicylates, except in the young, the old, and in people with hearing deficits for whom these symptoms are unreliable symptoms of salicylism. Patients treated with nonsteroidal antiinflammatory medications may have gastrointestinal complaints that can be avoided by dosing their medications at mealtimes or with antacids or carafate. Patients on hydroxychloroquine, gold, or cytotoxic agents should all be followed by a rheumatologist. Patients on hydroxychloroquine should have an ophthalmologic exam once every 6 months to look for early evidence of macular degeneration, a rare but devastating toxicity. Patients on intramuscular gold injections need to have a routine complete blood count, platelet count, and urinalysis with each gold injection, and patients on oral gold need these same laboratory checks monthly.

REFERENCES

Harris ED Jr: Pathogenesis of rheumatoid arthritis. In Kelley WN, Harris ED, Jr Ruddy S, Sledge CB (eds). *Textbooks of Rheumatology*. Third edition. WB Saunders, Philadelphia, 1989, pp 905–942.

Harris ED, Jr: The clinical features of rheumatoid arthritis. In Kelley WN, Harris ED Jr Ruddy S, Sledge CB (eds). *Textbook of Rheumatology*. Third edition. WB Saunders, Philadelphia, pp 943–981, 1989.

Harris ED Jr: Management of rheumatoid arthritis. In Kelley WN, Harris ED Jr Ruddy S, Sledge CB (eds). *Textbook of Rheumatology* Third edition. WB Saunders, Philadelphia, pp 982–992, 1989.

Utsinger PD, Zvaifler NJ, Ehrlich GE. (eds): *Arthritis: Etiology, Diagnosis, Management. Rheumatoid Arthritis.* JB Lippincott, Philadelphia, 1985.

11

Spondyloarthropathies

Spondyloarthropathies include at least six major rheumatic syndromes that have in common chronicity; male predominance; predilection for the spine (sacroiliitis and spondylitis) and, occasionally, peripheral joints; and extraarticular manifestations of rash, iritis, uveitis, conduction defects of the heart, aortic insufficiency, and apical fibrosis of the lungs; and are associated with HLA B27. These diseases also share a histological appearance of an inflammatory process with a predilection for the enthesis or areas where ligaments, tendons, and joint capsules join bone. The disorders include ankylosing spondylitis (AS), Reiter's syndrome (RS), psoriatic arthropathy (PsA), enteric arthropathy (with inflammatory bowel disease), juvenile chronic spondyloarthropathy, and reactive arthropathy (following dysentery or urethritis). The most common are ankylosing spondylitis and Reiter's syndrome. An understanding of these two syndromes and their management can be extrapolated to the less common and related syndromes.

CLINICAL PRESENTATION

The typical patient with ankylosing spondylitis presents with an insidious history of low back pain and stiffness which can be distinguished from garden-variety structural low back pain by the history and occasionally by physical examination early in the course. These characteristics are outlined in Table 4–6. The insidious onset is difficult to date but commonly occurs in late adolescence. The most important feature is that the symptoms are typically worse after prolonged inactivity (after arising or after prolonged periods of sitting), are improved by physical activity, and are not particularly helped by bed rest, unlike structural back pain, which is worse with spine use and is relieved by the supine position with the hips and knees flexed. Twenty percent of patients with ankylosing spondylitis have involvement of a peripheral joint before their spondylitis, and thus one should inquire about other joint pain that may have preceded back pain. The pattern of hand joint involvement can be useful to differentiate the spondyloarthropathies from other types of inflammatory arthritis. Spondyloarthropathies commonly cause *asymmetric* diffuse swelling of the digits (so-called sausage digits) or asymmetric joint involvement with distal interphalangeal joint predominance. An unusual presentation of spondyloarthropathies is one dominated by systemic symptoms of fatigue and general stiffness not well localized to the back. An occasional patient may present with only iritis and may not develop spondylitis until later.

The typical patient with Reiter's syndrome is a young male with iritis, urethritis, and skin lesions (balanitis or blennorrhagia keratoderma). In addition, patients may have painless oral ulcers or systemic symptoms. Reiter's syndrome may be confused with gonococcal arthritis, and one should consider the diagnosis of Reiter's syndrome in a patient who has persistent urethritis or arthritis and has been treated for a culture-negative gonococcal infection. Reiter's syndrome that follows dysentery from Yersinia, Shigella, Campylobac - ter, Salmonella, or Chlamydia is known as postdysenteric Reiter's syndrome. The typical patient is B27 positive and develops the syndrome within 2 weeks after dysentery. Treating the infection does not help the manifestations of Reiter's syndrome.

The natural history of ankylosing spondylitis is good, with most patients being functional, productive, and reasonably comfortable after many years of observation. Most patients will manifest which peripheral joints will be involved by 10 years of their disease, and patients who have early onset or who have hip, knee, shoulder, or ankle joints involved are likely to have worse function later on. Twenty-five percent of patients with ankylosing spondylitis develop iridocyclitis, usually unrelated to other evidence of inflammation, at some point in their course. This is managed with topical steroids. Patients should be warned about eye involvement and told to report it promptly. Delay in treatment may cause visual loss due to intraocular hypertension and synechiae and occasionally from band keratopathy. Patients with spondylitis may develop pulmonary fibrosis, particularly of the apical segments; aortic insufficiency, rarely requiring valve replacement; amyloid; fractures through calcified ligaments; heart conduction defects; meningoencephalitis; and peripheral neuropathies. The sacroiliitis of ankylosing spondylitis starts in the sacroiliac joints and with time obliterates the joints; it is associated with ascending calcification of the paraspinal ligaments from the lumbar to the cervical spine. Calcified ligaments can fracture and this is managed as an isolated incident with bed rest and conservative therapy. Spondylitis may also compromise the spinal canal, causing spinal stenosis.

The natural history of Reiter's syndrome is generally good, although some patients can have a chronic recurrent course. Their spondylitis, however, does not appear to be progessive. The principle limiting features in chronic Reiter's syndrome are the development of peripheral joint disease and, rarely, disabling iritis or balanitis.

DIAGNOSIS

The diagnosis of spondyloarthropathies is accomplished with a high index of suspicion, based principally on the history of inflammatory back pain and with confirmation by an x-ray of the sacroiliac joints. It is not important from a management point of view to distinguish between the various spondyloarthropathies early on, since management is the same. The diagnosis will eventually declare itself if other organ systems become involved. The x-ray confirmation can be done with a simple posteroanterior view of the pelvis, which also includes the hips. Additional views of the sacroiliac joints may make the diagnosis in some patients with subtle findings, but are generally not needed. Computed tomography or joint scans have been advocated, but there is tremendous overlap between normal individuals and those with sacroiliitis, and we do not recommend them.

The physical examination is not sensitive in the diagnosis of early spondyloarthropathy. The sacroiliac joints are quite deep and are inaccessible to direct examination. Mechanical causes of back pain can have the same physical findings. Measurement of spine mobility should be done, but unless the results are very abnormal, they are not as helpful for making a diagnosis as they are for following an individual patient. The two most common tests are Schober's test and chest expansion. Normal chest expansion should be more than 5 cm, and limited chest expansion in ankylosing spondylitis comes from involvement of costovertebral joints, which is usually a late finding. The Schober test measures the difference in distance between the line connecting the posterior iliac spines and a point 10 cm above and 5 cm below with the erect patient, and then in maximum forward flexion. However, the test can be abnormal in other causes of back pain that result in paraspinal muscle spasm or in patients with hip disease.

There are no specific laboratory abnormalities in ankylosing spondylitis or other spondyloarthropathies. The diagnosis of spondyloarthropathy rests mainly on history and x-ray. HLA B27 testing is marginally useful for diagnosis and does not affect prognosis or management in ankylosing spondylitis. In a patient with post-Yersinia Reiter's syndrome, the presence of B27 has prognostic value in that it increases the likelihood of developing syndesmophytes and sacroiliitis. In a few very problematic cases with a moderate rather than a low or high prior probability of having spondylitis, the test might be helpful. Spondyloarthropathies sometimes result in mild elevations of CPK and alkaline phosphatase. In general, the sedimentation rate does not reflect disease activity in spondyloarthropathies as well as in other inflammatory joint disease.

MANAGEMENT

In the spondyloarthropathies, the management of the arthritis or spondylitis centers on drug therapy and physical therapy. The spondyloarthropathies are more responsive to the indole-related nonsteroidal inflammatory drugs, which include indocin, tolectin, and phenylbutazone. Phenylbutazone should not be used, except briefly in flares, as it can cause agranulocytosis. The patient's symptoms, function, and spinal mobility are the chief things to follow. Laboratory evaluation is usually not more helpful than the patient's history or examination.

Physical therapy is a traditional component of managing spondylitis, although its effect has only been studied short term. The rationale for exercise is to maintain the spine in a position of most optimal function when and if fusion occurs. Exercise that can be incorporated into the patient's lifestyle is most likely to be followed over the long term of the disease. Swimming is an excellent way to extend the spine. Another is to have patients read the newspaper or watch television propped up on their elbows.

Other manifestations of both of these diseases can be treated conservatively. For instance, the conjunctivitis of Reiter's syndrome may be treated with topical steroids. Uveitis, more common in Reiter's syndrome, should be promptly evaluated by an ophthalmologist. Oral ulcers usually require no therapy, but if persistent may be treated with local cortisone preparations. Refractory Achilles tendonitis needs to be referred for more aggressive therapy.

REFERENCES

Blower PW, Griffin AJ: Clinical sacroiliac tests in ankylosing spondylitis and other causes of low back pain — 2 studies. Ann Rheum Dis 43:192–195, 1984.

Calin A (ed): *Spondyloarthropathies*. Grune and Stratton, New York, 1984.

Hawkins BR, Dawkins RL, Christiansen FT, Zilko initials: Use of the B27 test in the diagnosis of ankylosing spondylitis: A statistical evaluation. Arthritis Rheum 24:743–746, 1981.

Leirisalo M, et al.: Follow-up of Reiter's disease and reactive arthritis. Arthritis Rheum 25:249–290, 1982.

Roberts WN, Larson MG, Liang MH, Harrison RA, Barefoot J, Gall V, Clarke AK: Sensitivity of anthropometric techniques for long-term clinical trials in ankylosing spondylitis rehabilitation: Results of a natural experiment. Brit J. Rheum *28*:40–45, 1989.

Russell AS, Maksymowych W, LeClerc S: Clinical examination of the sacroiliac joints: A prospective study. Arthritis Rheum 24:1575–1581, 1981.

12 Bone Disorders (Osteoporosis, Paget's Disease)

Most primary bone disorders come to the attention of patients and their physicians by bone pain or as incidental findings on x-rays. Bone pain results from disturbances of or about the periosteum, the only innervated structure of the bone. This can come about as a result of stretching or inflammation. Patients with metabolic bone diseases and local disorders of bone may have structurally weakened bone, which may predispose them to microfractures (not always apparent on a conventional radiograph), or because abnormal bone shape alters the normal biomechanics of joint function and results in soft-tissue syndromes (chronic ligament or muscular strain). If local changes of Paget's disease or fractures from osteoporosis are near the joint, they may cause an incongruity of the joint surface, altered biomechanics, and pain.

DIAGNOSIS

There is no classical or typical history for bone pain, but some common presentations are diffuse discomfort unrelated to use, night pain, pain unresponsive to analgesics, or vague aches and pains without localizing findings. Fractures, especially in unusual places not clearly related to trauma or resulting from trivial trauma, should always make the physician think about the possibility of altered bone structure or bone disease. For example, young patients with a fractured rib after a cough may have osteoporosis from Cushing's Disease. Fractures of the foot without trauma could also suggest osteoporosis. Patients with underlying malignancy with unexplained pain, that is, without localizing physical findings, may have metastatic deposits, and if the x-ray is not diagnostic, a radionuclide scan needs to be done to identify osseous lesions. Persistant pain that is not explained by the examination should always be x-rayed and in some cases pursued with a bone scan. Very young and very old patients are at increased risk of having primary and metastatic bone tumors, respectively,

TABLE 12–1. CAUSES OF OSTEOPENIA

Osteoporosis	
Primary (idiopathic) or postmenopausal osteoporosis	
Senile or involutional	
Secondary osteoporosis	
Endocrinopathies	Cushing's syndrome
	Hyperparathyroidism
	Hyperthyroidism
	Ovarian failure, amenorrhea hypogonadism
Medications	Corticosteroid
	Heparin
	Methotrexate
	Anticonvulsants
Pregnancy	
Turner's syndrome	
Alcoholism	
Osteomalacia	
Dietary lack of vitamin D	
Gastrointestinal malabsorption	
Anticonvulsant therapy	
Chronic liver disease	
Chronic renal failure	
Renal tubular acidosis	
Hypophosphatemic osteomalacia (phosphate diabetes, vitamin-D-resistant osteomalacia)	
Vitamin-D-dependent osteomalacia	
Osteitis Fibrosa	
Primary and secondary hyperparathyroidism	
Malignancies	
Myeloma	
Metastatic bone disease	

which may frequently present as musculoskeletal pain in which the physical exam does not lead to the specific diagnosis.

The radiographic findings characteristic of diffuse metabolic disorders are either too little bone density or too much bone density. An x-ray of various bones ("bone survey") indicates whether the disorder is localized or generalized. *Osteopenia* is a generic term for decreased mineralized bone but is not a specific diagnosis (Table 12–1). In osteoporosis, the most common form of osteopenia, there is too little bone per volume of tissue for the age and sex of the individual. In osteoporosis, the proportion of bone mineral to bone matrix is normal and there is no detectable abnormality of bone composition. The bone matrix that is not mineralized is called *osteoid* and is present in excessive amounts in osteomalacia. Osteomalacia in adults is the same pathology as rickets in children. Osteitis fibrosa cystica, the bone lesion that occurs in some patients with hyperparathyroidism, is now rare. It is characterized by increased osteoclastic bone resorption and by proliferation of fibrous tissue in the bone. In most patients with osteitis fibrosa, the mineralized bone mass is less than normal. In some, bone formation appears to increase in compensation for the abnormal

TABLE 12–2. DIFFERENTIATING THE MAJOR CAUSES OF OSTEOPENIA

Type of Osteopenia	Serum Calcium	Serum Alkaline	Phosphate	Urine Calcium
Osteoporosis	Normal	Normal	Normal	Normal or elevated
Osteomalacia	Normal or low	Low	Elevated	Low
Osteitis fibrosa	Elevated	Elevated	Elevated	Elevated

Note exceptions: a) All serum chemistry may be normal in any form of osteopenia
b) In osteomalacia due to chronic renal failure, serum phosphate is increased

resorption, so there is no net bone loss. Some osteopenic patients with malignant disease, decreased bone per unit volume of tissue occurs with increased osteoclastic activity, while in others, evidence of abnormal osteoclastic activity is absent. In the latter group, it is thought that the tumor cells may be resorbing bone.

Table 12–2 gives a differential diagnosis of osteoporosis and osteomalacia. Evaluation of most of these disorders can be started by the generalist. For the more unusual forms, consultation may be required. The general sequence of evaluation begins with clinical suspicion that there is osteopenia. Since the x-ray only shows diminished bone mineral content when 40% to 50% of the calcium is already lost, conventional radiology is a relatively insensitive way to diagnose the condition. Dual-photon absorptometry, in particular, offers considerable advantages in measuring bone mass, and in longitudinal studies it is a strong predictor of osteoporotic fractures. Unfortunately, the technique cannot be recommended for general screening at this point. There is still considerable work to be done in standardization of the variety of machines before they can be generally recommended for the average practice and the results from different machines can be compared to one another. Bone biopsy is too invasive a procedure for routine evaluation but is frequently the single most informative test in nailing down a difficult diagnosis.

For the practitioner having thought of the possibility of metabolic bone disease, the next step is to assess whether the condition is generalized or localized, and to differentiated osteopenia and osteoporosis from osteomalacia. Short of a bone biopsy, serum chemistries may be very helpful. In malabsorption of vitamin D or dietary lack of vitamin D, serum calcium is low or low normal and the urine calcium is low. Since the major function of vitamin D and its metabolites is to stimulate calcium absorption from the gut, vitamin-D deficiency leads to decreased absorption, lowering serum calcium. In response to low serum calcium, the parathyroid glands secrete parathyroid hormone, which releases calcium from bone and increases alkaline phosphatase but decreases serum phosphate, since parathyroid hormone blocks phosphate resorption in the renal tubules and promotes phosphate loss in the urine.

The major goal in the differential diagnosis of osteopenia consists of distinguishing between osteoporosis and osteomalacia and then identifying those patients who have both. The first step is to rule out secondary forms of osteopenia. For this, a good history is the best test. For example, patients with a history of alcoholism, chronic liver disease, renal disease, malabsorption, or anticonvulsant therapy are quite likely to have osteomalacia or osteomalacia combined with osteoporosis.

If available, a determination of ionized calcium in the blood is desirable because this is a fraction of the total calcium that is regulated by hormones and controls cell metabolism. Most of the nonionized fraction of serum calcium is bound to plasma proteins, particularly albumin, and changes in these proteins may distort total serum calcium. For this reason, calcium must be interpreted in light of the total protein and albumin. Osteoporosis, in contrast, is usually accompanied by normal serum calcium, phosphate, and alkaline phosphatase. In osteomalacia, urine calcium is usually very low, less than 50 mg for 24 hours, as compared with a normal of 150 mg. Measurement of urinary creatinine provides an index of the adequacy of the urine collection and is used with the serum creatinine to give the creatinine clearance to assess renal function.

Endocrinopathies such as hyperthyroidism and Cushing's Syndrome can usually be suspected on clinical appearance, but disorders of calcium metabolism require specific testing. Serum protein electrophoresis, Bence Jones protein, and protein electrophoresis should be ordered, as myeloma is probably the most common malignancy associated with osteoporosis.

The serum 25-hydroxy vitamin D level very helpful to distinguish between osteoporosis and osteomalacia. A level below 10 mg/ml is seen in patients with a poor diet and/or malabsorption, and in those with liver disease associated with bile-duct obstruction. Low 25-hydroxy vitamin D suggests osteomalacia or, at least, that the patient is at risk for it.

There is only one pathognmonic finding in osteomalacia, and it only occurs in 5% to 10% of patients who have the disease. Radiographically, these individuals exhibit pseudofractures or Looser's lines, small areas of localized mineral loss from bones at sites where arteries enter bone, usually on the axillary side of the scapula, the pelvic brim, and the neck of the femur.

The urine and serum chemistry tests can sort out the major classes of disorders, and if the specific diagnosis cannot be made, referral is advised. Distinguishing osteoporosis and osteomalacia is necessary to devise the most specific and appropriate therapy. The usual treatment in both conditions is calcium and vitamin D, but the treatment can be toxic in patients with osteoporosis, who may get hypercalciuria and hypercalcemic on relatively small doses of vitamin D. For the patient with osteomalacia, larger doses are required and monitoring for hypercalciuria and hypercalcemia is mandatory.

MANAGEMENT OF OSTEOPOROSIS

When all of the above is said and done, 99% of patients with osteopenia will have osteoporosis and a negative workup, and the generalist will be faced with the issues of managing patients with primary osteoporosis.

Calcium replacement is the principal therapeutic option, except in two special cases. These special cases are osteomalacia and postmenopausal osteoporosis.

Estrogen given at the time of surgical or natural menopause, or in patients with established osteoporosis, maintains bone mass and decreases long bone

TABLE 12–3. RISK FACTORS FOR OSTEOPOROSIS

Menopause
Female
Sedentary
Smoking
White or Asian
Small frame
Malnutrition
Multiparity
Chronic obstructive lung disease
Steroid use

fractures. Theoretically, high-dose estrogen increase the risk of endometrial cancer, hypertension, thromboembolic disease, and cardiac disease, but the risk-benefit ratio for prescribing estrogens for preventing osteoporosis complications outweighs these. In practice, the doses of estrogen necessary for treatment of osteoporosis may actually retard the development of coronary artery disease in postmenopausal women and are not associated with an increased risk of thromboembolism in nonsmokers.

Prescribing estrogens has one side effect that many patients may not be able to tolerate — withdrawal bleeding. Many patients would prefer not to have menstrual bleeding for the rest of their lives. Cycling estrogens, that is, giving estrogens for 25 days out of the cycle and either nothing or a progestational agent for the remainder, allows the endometrium to be shed. Estrogen without a break, so to speak, develops hyperplastic endometrial tissue, which is thought to be a precursor to endometrial cancer and should be avoided. An unproven regimen gaining adherence in practice is simultaneous continuous use of 0.625 mg of conjugated estrogen (Premarin®) with 10 mg of progesterone daily. This combination provides estrogen while controlling endometrial hyperplasia and menstrual periods. How the efficacy and safety of this regimen compares to that of the traditional cycling regimen is unclear but is under active investigation.

The physician who writes prescriptions for estrogens should also be the one to follow up the potential side effects such as endometrial cancer.

A stepped approach to the management of osteoporosis involves prevention steps to maximize bone mass before puberty, particularly in high-risk individuals (Table 12–3); and at menopause, steps to prevent further bone loss and possibly to create new bone mass. The prevention of osteoporosis is best done early. This involves physical activity and probably diet. Physical activity stressing the long bone is important, as the principal stimulant of bone growth is gravity. Sunlight is important because it converts a precurser of vitamin D stored in the skin to an activated form. A good summer's worth of sunlight produces enough vitamin D to aid the body's economy nearly all the year. Calcium supplementation is necessary but the dose is debated. It should be between 1 to 2 g of elemental calcium a day. The average American diet gives roughly a half gram of calcium a day. One glass of milk, preferably skim, gives 250 mg of elemental calcium, which is the same dose available in one tablespoon of

Titralac® or one TUMS®. Balance studies suggest that in normal individuals, calcium carbonate is better absorbed than other forms of calcium, but it is not clear what difference this makes in practice. Calcium probably plays a minor role in maintaining bone mass in patients who are menopausal or who are already osteoporotic, but it is practically impossible not to permit or prescribe it and it probably does no harm. Calcium supplementation is contraindicated in those with a history of kidney stones and those who develop hypercalcuria after being started on calcium.

Supplemental vitamin D is recommended only for patients with a component of osteomalacia. Vitamin D is essential for normal calcium absorption and the requirement increases with age. People who do not receive enough sunlight (usually elderly house-bound women), who have poor diets, or who have disease in which there is malabsorption of vitamin D (small bowel diseases) might become vitamin-D deficient. No one should get more than 600 to 800 I.U. of vitamin D without clear indications or without monitoring for hypercalcemia. Prenatal vitamins often contain 400 IU of vitamin D.* Although the toxic does varies, 2 to 5000 I.U. a day can produce toxicity in some persons.

Steroid-induced osteoporosis requires different treatment and monitoring. The management or prevention of steroid-induced osteoporosis involves five to six times the amount of vitamin D used for osteoporosis and monitoring of urinary calcium to prevent nephrolithiasis and vitamin-D intoxication.

Sodium fluoride is the only medication that is shown to increase bone density in established osteoporosis but is still considered investigational, even after 20 years of investigation. The new bone formed by sodium fluoride may, however, be structurally inadequate and may even be more brittle than normal bone. Sodium fluoride without calcium and vitamin D can lead to the formation of osteoid that is not ossified, i.e., osteomalacia. The recommended dose of sodium fluoride is 20 mg twice a day. With this dose, many patients have gastric upset, arthralgias, or retain too much sodium, which can be a problem with patients who have difficulty handling salt, such as those with cirrhosis, renal disease, and congestive heart failure. We recommend that sodium fluoride be prescribed only in consultation with an endocrinologist or rheumatologist. Two regimens used for patients who have already experienced fracture include: daily calcitonin injections with oral fluoride, calcium, and vitamin D, or an estrogen/progesterone regimen with calcium fluoride and vitamin D. Consultation is also recommended.

In either case, a laboratory monitoring schedule should be aimed at detecting vitamin D toxicity (hypercalciuria) and proving that the regimen is actually doing something for bone mass, as there are responders and nonresponders to both of these regimens.

While other side effects and adverse outcomes are possible, or even likely (for example, gastrointestinal upset from oral fluoride), they are all events of which the patient would be aware. Therefore, failure of the regimen to do anything for

---

* 1 USP unit is equivalent to 1 IU, which is equivalent to 0.25 mg; 4 IU or USP units equals 1 mg of vitamin D.

bone mass and hypercalciuria (greater than 250 mg a day total calcium excretion in the urine), are the two outcomes in need of monitoring. Thus, baseline and quarterly determinations of 24-hour urine calcium are also required.

PAGET'S DISEASE

The most common cause of dense bone is Paget's disease. In general practice, Paget's disease is rarely symptomatic. Only 1% to 2% of people with radiographic Paget's disease have any clinical problem from the disease. Paget's disease is treated with diphosphonates, calcitonin, and mithramycin, all of which require experience for their management. The indications for referring Paget's patients for treatment are bone pain refractory to simple analgesics or antiinflammatory agents, spinal involvement with paraparesis, high-output cardiac failure, hearing loss, deformity of the long bone, and immobilization and hypercalcemia, which sometimes occur when a Paget's patient is bed rested. The most common error in management is misattribution of pain to Paget's disease when other factors are the cause.

REFERENCES

Consensus Conferences: Osteoporosis. JAMA 252:799–802, 1984.

Cummings SR, Black D: Should perimenopausal women be screened for osteoporosis? Ann Intern Med 104:817–823, 1986.

Harinck HIJ, Buvoet OLM, Vellenga JLR, et al.: Relation between signs and symptoms in Paget's disease of bone. Q J Med 58:133–151, 1986.

Louis V, Avioli: *The Osteoporotic Syndrome: Detection, Prevention, and Treatment.* Grune & Stratton, New York, 1988.

Riggs BL, Melton LJ: Involutional osteoporosis. N Engi J Med 26:1676–1684, 1986.

13

Systemic Lupus Erythematosus

Systemic lupus erythematosus (SLE) is a chronic inflammatory condition of unknown cause with protean clinical manifestations (Table 13–1). Presenting features can include fatigue, fever, and erythematous rash, polyarthralgia and arthritis, polyserositis, anemia, leukopenia, thrombocytopenia, renal, neurological, and cardiopulmonary disease (Table 13–2). Systemic lupus erythematosus affects primarily women, especially those of childbearing age and nonwhites. The prevalence for black females is nearly three times that for white females, and the disease appears to be more severe and associated with a higher mortality in blacks.

Systemic lupus erythematosus is in part a genetic disease in which female hormones appear to have an important facilitating or etiological role. Humoral immunological abnormalities must be important, since hypergammaglobulinemia and the presence of a panoply of autoantibodies to various cell constituents and hypocomplementemia are seen in most patients. Many patients with systemic lupus erythematosus also share immunological features such as decreased T cells and subsets of T cells, circulating immune complexes, and antilymphocyte autoantibodies as well.

Systemic lupus erythematosus can be fulminating and rapidly fatal, or a chronic and mild disease. With the advent of sensitive serologic tests, many cases are diagnosed that are mild with an irregular course over many years with periods of complete or nearly complete remission. In contrast to the early understanding of the disease, it is no longer thought of as a uniformly fatal disease. In fact, most individuals live fairly normal lives despite their symptoms. The chief reasons for death are related to infectious complications, perhaps as a result of aggressive immunosuppressive therapy, renal failure, central nervous system involvement, or, late in the course, atherosclerotic complications of steroid treatment and immune complex damage to endothelium, including coronary artery disease and stroke.

An important and "treatable" cause of lupus is a lupus syndrome caused by a

TABLE 13–1. CLINICAL MANIFESTATIONS OF SYSTEMIC LUPUS ERYTHEMATOSUS

Constitutional (fatigue, malaise, fever, weight loss)
Raynaud's Phenomenon
Cutaneous
Malar rash
Discoid rash
Photosensitivity
Oral ulcers
Alopecia
Vasculitis
Rash, other (urticarial, bullous, maculopapular subacute cutaneous, panniculitis)
Ocular
conjunctivitis/episcleritis
sicca
Cardiopulmonary
pleurisy/pleural effusions
pericarditis
myocarditis
Libman–Sacks endocarditis
pneumonitis
interstitial fibrosis/pulmonary hypertension
Gastrointestinal
anorexia, nausea, abdominal pain
vasculitis
sterile peritonitis
Musculoskeletal
arthralgia/myalgias
nonerosive polyarthritis
myositis
Hematologic
anemia
hemolytic anemia
neutropenia
lymphopenia
thrombocytopenia
lupus anticoagulant
lymphadenopathy
splenomegaly
Renal
glomerulonephritis
membranous
focal glomerulitis
nephrotic syndrome
Central Nervous System
organic brain syndrome
cognitive
psychosis
peripheral neuropathy
seizure
stroke, transverse myelitis

variety of drugs or *drug-induced lupus*. Unlike patients with idiopathic lupus, patients with the drug-induced lupus syndrome have more serositis and rarely have brain or kidney involvement. Antibodies against native double-stranded DNA are absent; antihistone antibodies are often present. The clinical picture is dominated by arthralgias, pleurisy, pericarditis, and pulmonary effusions — much like the picture of lupus in the older patient. Medications implicated in

TABLE 13–2. FREQUENCIES OF PRESENTATIONS OF SYSTEMIC LUPUS ERYTHEMATOSUS

Arthralgias, arthritis	27%
Systemic (fever, weight loss, fatigue)	25
Multisystem disease	22
Skin rash	20
Other (serositis, hematologic)	6

TABLE 13–3. DRUGS ASSOCIATED WITH DRUG-INDUCED LUPUS

Definite	Possible	Unlikely
Hydralazine	Diphenylhydantoin	Griseofulvin
Procainamide	Chlorpromazine	Phenylbutazone
Isoniazid	Methyldopa	Oral contraceptives
	Penicillamine	Gold salts
	Quinidine	Sulfonamide
	Propylthiouracil	Penicillin
	Lithium carbonate	

TABLE 13–4. FEATURES DISTINGUISHING BETWEEN SPONTANEOUS SYSTEMIC LUPUS ERYTHMATOSUS AND DRUG-INDUCED LUPUS

	Spontaneous SLE (%)	Drug-Induced Lupus (%)
Constitutional symptoms (fever, malaise, myalgia)	80	50
Arthralgia and arthritis	90	95
Pleuropericarditis	50	50
Hepatomegaly	25	25
Skin rash (all types)	75	10–20
Discoid lesions	20	0
Malar rash	40	2
Renal involvement	50	5
CNS involvement	30	0
Serologic abnormalities ANA	95	95
Anti-RNP	40	20
Anti-Sm	20	0
Anti-N-DNA	90	0
Antihistone	25	90

this disorder are given in Table 13–3. Distinguishing features of systemic lupus erythematosus and drug-induced lupus are outlined in Table 13–4. These features cannot be used to absolutely diagnose the condition and any drug that can be stopped should be stopped.

The most common culprits are hydralazine and procainamide. Antinuclear antibodies develop in over half of the patients after 2 years of taking hydralazine, but only 1 out of 7 have a significant titer, and only 4% develop the clinical syndrome of systemic lupus erythematosus. Autoantibodies may be seen in 50% of individuals taking procainamide for several months, and about one-half of these subjects eventually develop a lupuslike syndrome. With isoniazid, 20% of the patients develop autoantibodies, but it is rare for drug-induced lupus to occur.

DIAGNOSIS

Systemic lupus erythematosus should be considered in any patient who has a systemic illness in which multiple organ systems are involved and who has an antinuclear antibody (ANA) in a significant titer. A positive antinucler antibody does not make the diagnosis of lupus, and a rare patient with lupus will not have a positive antinuclear antibody. Of the precipitins to antinuclear antibodies, the antibody to double-stranded DNA and to Sm are the most specific for lupus. Other diseases can mimic systemic lupus erythematosus, and these include rheumatoid arthritis, scleroderma, drug-induced systemic lupus erythematosus, polyarteritis nodosa, and other systemic vasculitis, chronic active hepatitis, and drug reactions. Common diseases such as *Acne rosacea* (malar distribution) and fibrositis or bursitis also mimic systemic lupus erythematosus. Systemic lupus erythematosus is, however, a clinical diagnosis, and some patients, particularly early in the course, may not demonstrate all features or even have a positive antinuclear antibody. However, 95% of patients do have a positive antinuclear antibody; antinuclear antibodies that are negative after a year of symptoms will remain so.

The common presentations of lupus are outlined in Table 13–2. Constitutional symptoms, fever, fatigability, and weight loss are often insidious and only a few or one organ system may be involved in the beginning, which makes the diagnosis difficult. Joint involvement is the most common manifestation of systemic lupus erythematosus and may precede other system involvement by years.

TREATMENT

There is no cure for systemic lupus erythematosus, but the vast majority of patients can be managed with a minimum of medications and may expect to have an impaired but reasonably normal life. The object is to control flare-ups and to treat major organ involvement such as brain, kidney, cardiopulmonary, and hematological manifestations. Patients without major organ involvement may be disabled by arthralgias and fatigue, and these symptoms should be manged without glucocorticoids. Arthralgias, arthritis, myalgias, fever, and mild serositis can usually be treated with nonsteroidal antiinflammatory drugs, including salicylates, even though they may have slightly more toxicity than in patients without the disease. Subjective fatigue can be improved with aerobic conditioning. Exercise usually does not make quiescent joint symptoms flare. The cutaneous manifestations of lupus, including discoid lesions, and joint symptoms, respond to antimalarials. Hydroxycloroquine in doses of 400 mg a day usually improves these mainfestations in a few weeks. Antimalarials may cause retinal toxicity and less frequently rash, myopathy, and neuropathy, and thus a patient who is maintained on this medication must have regular retinal examinations to look for the earliest signs of ocular toxicity. Cutaneous lupus is also treated with topical glucocorticoids, and for those with severe and disfiguring lesions, systemic glucocorticoids should be considered. Sun exposure may induce flares of joint, visceral, and skin disease in about a third of patients with lupus. These patients should avoid the maximum ultraviolet radiation occurring during the midday and should use sunscreens with an sun protection factor rating of 15 or higher. If glucocorticoids are considered, referral is advisable since they are effective, but in long-term high doses, they have considerable side effects. The questions of if and when to stop and how to taper require some experience.

Life-threatening and disabling manifestations of lupus are usually treated with glucocorticoids in a dose of 1 mg/kg body weight/day. Moderate manifestations often respond to 30 mg/day. Every other day corticosteroid regimens usually fail. Some clinicians will not taper the last 5 to 10 mg of prednisone, no matter how well the patient is doing, for fear of bringing on an exacerbation. Antimalarials may be used to maintain a remission and some evidence suggest that they are steroid-sparing. The usual approach in starting steroids is to give them in divided doses until the disease has been controlled for several days and to consolidate the dose to a once-a-day dose in the morning. Obtaining a battery of laboratory and immunological tests is helpful to characterize the patient and to find other markers of disease activity that can be used in following the patient and in making decisions on steroid taper. Steroids bring a host of problems, including iatrogenic Cushing's disease, weight gain, hypertension, increased susceptibility to infection, capillary fragility, acne, hirsutism, accelerated osteoporosis, ischemic necrosis of bone, cataracts, glaucoma, diabetes mellitus, myopathy, hyperglycemia, and central nervous system effects, including insomnia, mania, and psychosis. Thus, every patient who is on steroids should be considered a high-risk patient, and general health maintenance should be provided. Eye evaluation should be done periodically. Skin and dental hygiene are also important. Infections should be identified early and treated promptly. Immunizations with influenza and pneumococcal vaccine are safe and are effective in patients with stable disease. Supplemental calcium, 1500 mg daily, with vitamin D, 50,000 units weekly, in patients with normal 24-hour urine calcium and normal serum calcium may help maintain bone mass.

The use of other cytotoxic agents such as azathioprine and cyclophosphamide in addition to steroids is required for some desperate situations. Efficacy, particularly of azathioprine or of cyclophosphamide in situations other than glomerulonephritis, is debated. In lupus nephritis, particularly with rapidly progressive glomerulonephritis and for patients with biopsies that show scarring or evidence of current activity, cyclophosphamide probably is effective. These agents should not be started without consultation.

Patients should be referred if the clinical presentation is not diagnostic, if steroid or immunosuppressive therapy is considered, if a patient is not responding to conservative management, or if a patient has renal, cardiac, or central nervous system involvement.

REFERENCES

Fries JF, Holman HR: *Systemic Lupus Erythematosus.* WB Saunders, Philadelphio, 1975.

Lahita RG (ed): *Systemic Lupus Erythematosus.* John Wiley & Sons, New York, 1987.

Ropes MW: *Systemic Lupus Erythematosus.* Harvard University Press, Cambridge, MA, 1986.

Schur PH (ed): *The Clinical Management of Systemic Lupus Erythematosus.* Grune and Stratton, Orlando, FL, 1983.

Wallace DJ Dubois EL, Quismorio, FP Jr, Klinenberg JR (ed): *Dubois' Lupus Erythematosus.* Lea & Febiger, Philadelphia, 1987.

14

Raynaud's Phenomenon and Associated Diseases

Raynaud's phenomenon is reversible pallor from vasospasm of the fingers, hand, toes, nose, earlobe, or tongue precipitated by cold or emotion. The reaction is episodic and may be accompanied by numbness or pain. The syndrome is classically described as a triphasic response with blanching white color, usually clearly demarcated from the rest of the digit, followed by cyanosis and then rubor as reperfusion takes place. A distinction is made between Raynaud's phenomenon, which occurs with or is an early manifestation of a connective tissue disease and Raynaud's disease, which occurs much more commonly as an isolated condition.

Many patients with Raynaud's phenomenon and many without it complain of having cold hands or color changes of the hands. Since there is no blood test, standardized bedside diagnostic tests, or even clinical criteria for Raynaud's phenomenon, the history is the primary basis for diagnosis.

The *episodic* nature and pallor are the two critical historical features. Rubor and cyanosis are nonspecific symptoms. Cyanosis, for instance, occurs with vasoconstriction, secondary to cooling. Rubor is seen in some but not all patients with vascular diseases as the result of reactive hyperemia after the blood flow is reestablished. Pallor alone without cyanosis or rubor is enough to make a diagnosis. Another feature that distinguishes Raynaud's phenomenon from cold extremities or acrocyanosis is a sharp area of demarcation from the rest of the digit.

Even in a referral practice, only 5% of patients with Raynaud's phenomenon develop a connective tissue disease. Many rheumatic diseases can be associated with Raynaud's phenomenon (scleroderma, CREST, systemic lupus erythematosus, mixed connective tissue disease, dermatomyositis, or rheumatoid arthritis), but the most important are scleroderma and related disorders.

Systemic sclerosis is a generalized disorder of connective tissue characterized by fibrosis and degenerative changes in the skin, synovium, digital arteries, and small arteries of internal organs, most notably, the esophagus, intestine, lungs,

TABLE 14–1. THE SCLERODERMAS

I. Progressive systemic slerosis (PSS)
   A. PSS with diffuse scleroderma — symmetric, diffuse involvement of the skin (scleroderma) affecting trunk, face, proximal and distal portions of the extremities; relatively early appearance of disease of the esophagus, intestine, heart, lungs and kidney
   B. CREST syndrome — relatively limited involvement of the skin, often confined to the fingers and face; prominence of sclerodactyly, telangiectasis, and prolonged appearance of distinctive internal manifestations (including severe pulmonary arterial hypertension and biliary cirrhosis)
   C. Overlap syndromes, including sclerodermatomyositis and mixed connective tissue disease
II. Eosinophilic fasciitis
III. Congenital fascial dystrophy
IV. Localized dystrophy
   A. Morphea
   B. Linear scleroderma
   C. Scleroderma en coup de sabre, with or without facial hemiatrophy
V. Chemically induced conditions
   A. Vinylchloride
   B. Pentazocine-induced fibrosis
   C. Bleomycin-induced fibrosis
   D. L-5-hydroxytryptophan and carbidopa
VI. Digital sclerosis and joint contractures associated with juvenile-onset diabetes mellitus
VII. Diseases with skin changes resembling scleroderma
   A. Edematous
      1. Scleroderma related to diabetes mellitus
      2. Scleromyxedema (papular mucinosis)
   B. Indurative and/or atrophic
      1. Lichen sclerosus et atrophicus
      2. Porphyria cutanea tarda
      3. Acromegaly
      4. Myeloma-associated and primary amyloidosis
      5. Skin thickening associated with plasma-cell neoplasia and peripheral polyneurophagy
      6. Carcinoid syndrome
   C. Paraneoplastic palmar fasciitis occurring with ovarian, breast, and colon carcinoma.

heart, and kidney. The spectrum of disease ranges from restricted skin involvement confined to the face and hands to widespread skin involvement with visceral involvement. The cause is unknown. Scleroderma skin is shiny, waxy, and without normal wrinkles. A number of diseases, all rare, may cause tight skin (Table 14–1). Eosinophilic fasciitis, though rare, is one condition that seems to respond to steroids.

Clinically, scleroderma appears as focal or generalized areas of skin change. Early scleroderma, has a nonpitting, swollen, puffy appearance. The patient describes difficulty with taking off rings and lack of normal mobility. These are subtle changes that may only be apparant to the patient. The demarcation at which the puffy skin makes the transition to normal skin is gradual. The fact that there is no pitting edema or focal swelling over joints or tendons suggests the dermatological nature of the condition.

As the disease progresses, the involved skin becomes bound down and shiny, with noticeable loss of wrinkles and skinfolds. The scleroderma facies is characterized by a pinched, immobile expressionless face and a narrowed oral aperture. Changes of hyperpigmentation, telangiectases, subcutaneous calcifications, and atrophy of the distal digital tufts may occur.

Scleroderma involvement is ascertained by seeing whether the skin can be picked up with the thumb and the index finger. Systemic sclerosis starts distally in the digits, results in sclerodactyl, and "marches" towards the torso. The earliest manifestation is the inability to pinch the skin between the distal interphalangeal and proximal interphalangeal joints.

Early scleroderma or sclerodactyly is a problem for the generalist and the specialist. Criteria to predict which patients will have progressive skin or internal organ involvement are under active study. Patients with Raynaud's phenomenon at risk of developing systemic sclerosis may be identified at an early stage by distinctive nailfold capillary changes, which can be visualized with a dissection microscope or a 30 to 40x ophthalmoscope lens. The keratinized layer is rubbed with mineral oil to make it translucent enough for visualization of capillary loops. Patients who have Raynaud's phenomenon for 5 years and do not develop signs of systemic illnesses probably will not do so, but even 20 years of follow-up is not an absolute guarantee if there are any nailfold capillary changes.

DIAGNOSIS OF RAYNAUD'S PHENOMENON

The principal task in evaluating Raynaud's phenomenon is to determine whether it is isolated, associated, or caused by other diseases or exposures. Table 14–2 shows the differential diagnosis of Raynaud's phenomenon, but the vast majority of patients with the disease can be evaluated quite simply. The intensity or type of evaluation (Table 14–3) depends on whether the disease occurs in all the extremities or is symmetric, which suggests a systemic cause; is isolated to one extremity, which suggests a regional neurovascular cause such as the thoracic outlet syndrome or old cold injury; the age and sex of the patient; and whether the patient is sick.

Patients who are young, who look and feel well, and who have had Raynaud's phenomenon for less than 5 years need only a complete history, physical, and follow-up. Patients over age 40, people who look sick or who have symptoms referable to other organs, or those who have the disease in a severe enough form to interfere with function require more thorough evaluation.

Treatment of Raynaud's phenomenon begins with measures of avoidance and drug and surgical therapies. These patients should avoid cigarette smoke, cold, and beta blockers. The body temperature is important, and wearing a hat and vest can be beneficial. Waving the involved arm can be helpful. Biofeedback training works when available. Calcium-channel blockers, including nifidepine and diltiazem have been used with success. Intraarticular reserpine probably does not work. Sympathectomy works but patients often suffer relapse between 18 and 24 months afterwards. Plasmapheresis has been tried and can be useful when there is a measurable immune complex or cryoglobulin circulating that can be removed; it is usually ineffective otherwise.

TABLE 14–2. CONDITIONS ASSOCIATED WITH RAYNAUD'S PHENOMENON (SECONDARY RAYNAUD'S PHENOMENON)

Small-Vessel Disease

Idiopathic
- systemic sclerosis
- systemic lupus erythematosus
- rheumatoid arthritis
- dermatomyositis — polymyositis
- vasculitis

Vibration, chronic (i.e., jack hammers, chain saw)
Cold injury
Primary pulmonary hypertension

Large-Vessel Disease

Arteriosclerosis
Prinzmetal angina
Thoracic outlet syndromes
Thromboangiitis obliterans

Intravascular (Cyanosis without Blanching)

Cryoglobulinemias
Cold agglutinins
Polycythemia

Drug or Toxin Associated

Beta blockers
Ergots
Bleomycin
Cisplatin
Vincristine/vinblastine
Nicotine
Pseudoephedrine polyvinylchloride

Hormonal

Hypothyroidism
Estrogen-progesterone
Pheochromocytoma

TABLE 14–3. RAYNAUD'S PHENOMENON — RED FLAGS

Sign or Symptom	Significance
Systemic symptoms	Rheumatic disorder Paraneoplastic syndrome
Sclerodactyly, bilateral	Scleroderma
Compromised skin nutrition	Impending gangrene
Advancing scleroderma	Organ involvement
Abnormal nailfold capillaries	Scleroderma, sle polymyositis
Hypertension	Organ involvement

If the phenomen is established, look carefully for sclerodactyly or skin changes that suggest scleroderma. Patients with sclerodactyly or who are ill need to be thoroughly evaluated to determine end-organ involvement and function. The principal organs of concern are the lungs (chest x-ray, pulmonary function testing including diffusion capacity), kidney, liver, and joints. Most organ involvement is suggested by a review of systems, but everybody should have, as a basic workup, an antinuclear antibody (ANA), a urinalysis, an erythrocyte sedimentation rate, and a complete blood count and serum creatinine or BUN. An antinuclear antibody is done because Raynaud's phenomenon can be a manifestation of lupus, and testing for antinuclear antibodies is the most sensitive indication of that. Erythrocyte sedimentation rate elevation, similarly, indicates an inflammatory condition that might require further workup.

Anybody with Raynaud's phenomenon who has other organ involvement could have secondary Raynaud's phenomenon and should be referred to a rheumatologist at some point.

Certain clinical features are extremely important (Table 14–3). Hypertension, renal involvement, or progressive sclerodactyly are ominous signs and symptoms, herald an impending crisis with scleroderma, and should be referred for aggressive management. Anticentromere and antibody to Scl 70, new antibodies, are useful for classifying scleroderma and are frequently positive in patients with positive antinuclear antibodies and have prognostic value. The two examinations that should be done at every office visit of a patient with Raynaud's phenomenon or sclerodactyly are a) examination of the skin for progression of tight skin and b) a blood pressure measurement as a screen for renal involvement.

REFERENCES

Fitzgerald O, Hess EV, O'Connor GT, Spencer–Green G: Prospective study of the evolution of Raynaud's phenomenon. Am J Med 84:718–726, 1988.

Fritzler MJ, Ayer LM: Anticentromere antibodies. Clinical and biological significance. J Rheum 9:489–490, 1982.

Gerbracht DD, Steen VD, Ziegler GL, Medsger TA, Rodnan GP: Evolution of primary Raynaud's phenomenon (Raynaud's disease) to connective tissue disease. Arthritis Rheum 28:87–92, 1985.

Kenik JG, Maricg HR, Bole GG: Blind evalution of the diagnostic specificity of nailfold capillary microscopy in the connective tissue diseases. Arthritis Rheum 24:885–891, 1981.

Priollet P, Vayssairat M, Housset E: How to classify Raynaud's phenomenon: Long-term follow-up study of 73 cases. Am J Med 83:494–498, 1987.

15 Vasculitis Syndromes

Vasculitis is a term applied to a large number of syndromes whose common feature is inflammation and necrosis of blood vessels. (Table 15–1). The histopathology is characterized by findings that include polymorphonuclear, mononuclear, or giant cells and varying degrees of fibrinoid necrosis, disruption of normal vascular architecture, or endothelial proliferation. The clinical manifestations depend on which vessels are affected and to what degree. Multiple clinical/pathological classification schemes have been devised based on histopathology or which vessels are affected, and the American College of Rheumatology is in process of devising diagnostic criteria. These systems are most useful for retrospective studies and characterizing subjects for analysis. Clinical studies suggest considerable overlap in both histology and clinical presentations. Table 15–2 gives a classification scheme based on dominant organ-system manifestation and therapy. The pathological appearance of the lesions is helpful in a) determining whether arteries or veins are principally affected, b) whether the process is more active or more "burned out," the latter implying irreversibility, c) deciding whether the patient needs prednisone and/or an immunosuppressive agent such as cyclophosphamide, d) the extent of involvement, and d) whether the lesions are more granulomatous or angiitic.

The possibility of vasculitis should be considered when there is palpable purpura, multisystem disease, and constitutional symptoms, or when a vascular event such as stroke or claudication occurs in an unusual clinical setting (i.e., stroke in a young woman). Fever, weight loss, and night sweats occur in 90% of patient with vasculitis. Athralgias, arthritis, and myalgias are also seen. Abdominal pain without focal findings, and often with postprandial pain, may be the result of mesenteric arteritis or sterile peritonitis. Renal involvement occurs in about a half of patients with systemic vasculitis and may be evidenced by an active urinary sediment. Skin lesions are highly specific for vasculitis and, depending on the vessel size involved, may present with splinter hemorrhages (small vessel), palpable purpura (medium size), ulcer, or gangrene (small vessel),

TABLE 15–1. THE SYSTEMIC VASCULITIDES

Systemic necrotizing vasculitis
Polyartertitis nodosa
Rheumatoid vasculitis
Allergic granulomatosis (Churg-Strauss)
Giant-cell arteritis
Temporal arteritis
Takayasu's arteritis
Hypersensitivity vasculitis
Schonlein–Henoch purpura
Leukocytoclastic vasculitis
Serum sickness (immunizations, drugs, streptokinase, etc.)
Vasculitis associated with rheumatoid arthritis and systemic lupus erythmatosus
Subacute bacterial endocarditis
Vasculitis associated with malignancies
Essential cryoglobulinemia with vasculitis
Wegener's granulomatosis
Lymphomatoid granulomatosis
Thromboangiitis obliterans (Buerger's disease)
Goodpasture's syndrome
Kawasaki's disease (acute febrile mucocutaneous lymph node syndrome)

Neurological manifestations may range from an isolated peripheral neuropathy to stroke syndromes (cerebrovasculor accident, transverse myelitis, cranial neuropathy) to diffuse brain involvement.

DIAGNOSIS

In an illness with multisystem organ involvement and constitutional systems, vasculitis, sepsis, neoplasm, or emboli (cholesterol, infected emboli such as acute or subacute bacterial endocarditis), left atrial myxoma, and connective tissue disease are the diagnostic possibilities. Making a general working diagnosis of vasculitis and following a patient with vasculitis should be in the generalist's repertoire, but consultation is almost always required. The physician needs to methodically evaluate the organ systems involved by history, physical exam, and laboratory in each case (Table 15–3). Once the extent and severity of involvement has been established, the physician must hospitalize the patient, an emergent evaluation by subspecialists is required, or it must be determined whether the patient is stable. Suspected vasculitis should be referred, or it must be determined whether the patient is stable. Suspected vasculitis should be referred for more specific diagnosis and treatment.

The most incisive and diagnostic test in suspected vasculitis is a biopsy of the affected tissue/organ. This should always be done before starting therapy with corticosteroids or other immunosuppressive agents. Sites with high yield include skin lesions, sural nerve identified by conduction abnormalities, tender muscle or blind muscle biopsy, tender epididymal nodules in suspected polyarteritis nodosa, kidney when clinical nephritis exists, nasopharyngeal biopsy in a suspected Wegener's granulomatosis, and the temporal artery when the temporal

TABLE 15–2. CLASSIFICATION OF VASCULITIS

	Periarteritis Nodosa	Allergic Granulomatosis (Churg–Strauss)	Wegener's Granulomatosis	Leucocytoclastic Angiitis	Takayasu's and Giant-Cell Arteritis
Involved blood vessels	Muscular arteries, occasional arterioles	Muscular arteries, adjacent veins, occasional arterioles	Arteries, arterioles, venules, some capillaries	Arterioles, venules, capillaries	Large and medium arteries
Histology	Necrotizing inflammation, acute and healing lesions	Necrotizing inflammation, acute and healing lesions, giant cells	Necrotizing inflammation, granulomas, acute and healing lesions	Necrotizing inflammation, lesions in same stage	Inflammation without necrosis, giant cells
Clinical involvement	Widespread, branching points of arteries, lungs not involved	Widespread; lungs frequently involved	Upper and lower respiratory tract	Skin, serosa, glomeruli	Large arteries and branches

TABLE 15–3. INITIAL EVALUATION FOR SUSPECTED VASCULITIS

Clinical

Skin
- petechia
- purpura
- hives
- nodules

Eyes
- iritis
- episcleritis
- ischemic optic disc
- papilledema
- cytoid bodies

Enteric
- ulcers
- septal perforation
- sinus involvement

Respiratory
- lymphadenopathy

Chest
- rales

Cardiovascular
- ectopy
- pericardial effusion
- bruits

Abdominal
- hepatosplenomegaly
- bruit

Laboratory
- hematocrit
- hemoglobin
- white blood count
- differential
- platelet estimate or count
- erythrocyte sedimentation rate
- urine analysis
- serum creatinine
- aklaline phosphatase
- creatine phosphokinase
- SGOT, SGPT
- chest x-ray
- electrocardiogram
- stool for occult blood

artery is clinically abnormal in suspected giant cell or temporal arteritis. In suspected polyarteritis nodosa, celiac axis arteriography may be diagnostic.

TREATMENT

The diagnosis and treatment of vasculitis is best left in the hands of someone experienced in management, since the conditions are rare and treatment recommendations are in flux. Some generalizations are useful, however. Isolated skin or peripheral nervous system involvement can be watched, whereas systemic vasculitis involving major organs, brain, lung, heart, and kidney requires aggres-

TABLE 15–4. MEDICAL TREATMENT OF VASCULITIS

Options	Disease
Expectant	Leukocytoclastic angiitis Henoch–Schonlein purpura Serum sickness
Corticosteriods	Temporal arteritis Takayasu's arteritis Allergic granulomatosis (Churg–Strauss) Polyarteritis nodosa
Corticosteroids and cyclophosamide	Wegener's granulomatosis Some polyarteritis nodosa Some rheumatoid vasculitis

TABLE 15–5. CRITERIA FOR REFERRAL

Suspected vasculitis
Neurologic involvement
Abdominal pain
Renal involvement
Cardiopulmonary involvement

sive treatment. In systemic vasculitis, treatment consists of supportive care, steroids (high dose), and, in specific forms, an alkylating agent (Table 15–4). In cutaneous vasculitis when no systemic vasculitis exists, either primary or secondary, the patient should be followed only. Potential triggers, principally drugs, should be stopped. Infection must always be considered. The demonstrably steroid-sensitive vasculitis syndromes include giant-cell arteritis, Takayasu's disease and systemic lupus erythmatosus vasculitis. The syndromes requiring alkylating agents (usually cyclophosphamide) include Wegener's granulomatosis and some forms of polyarteritis nodosa and rheumatoid vasculitis. These groups can overlap and some supposedly steroid-sensitive forms will require the addition of an alkylating agent for adequate control.

The prognosis of patients with vasculitis varies widely. The prognosis of hypersensitivity angiitis (leucocytoclastic angiitis) without systemic invdvement is generally good, with most patients making a full recovery over several months. Giant-cell arteritis may be active for months to years, with a median of 7 months. Polyarteritis nodosa usually runs its course over months to years. Death occurs in 20% despite treatment and is due to myocardial infarction, hypertensive disease, or progressive renal failure. Patients with Wegener's granulomatosis respond to cyclophosphamide within 2 to 4 weeks of therapy but can die of renal or pulmonary involvement. Some patients with rheumatoid vasculitis or polyarteritis nodosa may need cyclophosamide, as well, for the best results.

Patients who survive acute vasculitis of medium- to large-sized vessels are at risk of developing late arteriosclerotic vascular disease (stroke, coronary artery disease) and meticulous attention should be given to modifying other risk factors (smoking, lipids, hypertension); these patients should probably receive low-dose aspirin.

In summary, the hallmark of vasculitis is multisystem involvement. The most important decision to make is whether or not the patient is sick and requires immediate hospitalization because of organ system involvement or can be worked up in a more leisurely manner. Secondly, a directed work up should be done to characterize the organ systems, particularly the skin, the neurological, cardiovascular, pulmonary, and gastrointestinal systems. Thirdly, early referrals for definitive diagnosis are suggested (Table 15–5).

REFERENCES

Cupps T, Fauci AS: In LH Smith Jr (ed). *The Vasculitides. Major Problems in Internal Medicine*. WB Saunders, Philadelphia 1981.

Fauci AS, Haynes BF, Katz P: The spectrum of vasculitis. Clinical pathologic, immunologic, and therapeutic considerations. Ann Intern Med 89:660, 1978.

Hunder GG, Lie JT: The Vasculitides. Clin Cardiovasc Dis 13:261, 1983.

Lichtenstein LM, Fauci AS: *Current Therapy In Allergy, Immunology, and Rheumatology-3.* BC Decker, Philadelphia, 1988.

16 Myopathy Syndromes

The most common complaints referable to the muscles are cramps, weakness, myalgias (aches and pains), and the occasional patient with isolated muscle enzyme elevation. These problems (Table 16–1) can be sorted out effectively by a good history and an exam looking for signs of abnormal muscle function. The types of muscle complaints seen in primary care practice are almost always benign and self-limited. With reasonable care, serious forms of myopathy (Table 15–2) can be excluded without difficulty.

HISTORY AND DIAGNOSIS

The history gets at the following points:

- Whether symptoms are periodic, constant, a progressive
- The distribution of the symptoms (bulbar, proximal, distal, or general)
- Whether symptoms are use-related
- To distinguish weakness from asthenia or general lassitude.

Constant weakness due to loss of muscle power is that which is unchanged from day to day, week to week, and within a day. Weakness due to primary muscle disorders or from metabolic causes such as myasthenia gravis are quite variable and are often related to ambient temperature (i.e., heat makes almost all forms of myopathies worse) or to the use of the specific muscles. An absolutely constant weakness suggests a neurological cause such as peripheral neuropathy, cord lesion, or stroke. In the patient with complaints of consistent weakness with no variability in symptoms either related to use or to the ambient temperature in which there are no objective findings of weakness, a functional cause should be sought.

The distribution of the weakness and cramps is useful in distinguishing syndromes. A peripheral local asymmetric weakness is likely to be neurological. Proximal, symmetric weakness is seen in almost all forms of both primary and

TABLE 16–1. MUSCLE SYNDROMES

Generalized Weakness: Acute (days) or subsequent (weeks), usually with no atrophy

Myasthenia gravis
Muscle weakness — Drug-induced
- Beta blockers
- diphenylhydantoin
- procainamide
- antibiotics — karamycin, gentamycin, colistin, tetracycline, neomycin, polymyxin, streptomycin
- corticosteroids
- hydroxychloroquine
- cimetidine
- penicillamine
- ethanol
- lithium
- toluene
- plaquenil
- lovastatin

Acute Polio, Idiopathic Polyneuritis, or Other Polyneuropathy

- Polymyositis and dermatomyositis
- Acute paroxysmal myoglobinuria
- "Alcoholic" myopathy
- First attack of episodic weakness (see below)
- Botulism
- Organophosphate poisoning
- Diabetic neuropathy syndromes including diabetic amyotrophy

Generalized Weakness Subacute or Chronic (months to years; usually with atrophy)

Progressive muscular dystrophy
- Duchenne type
- facioscapulohumeral type
- limb girdle types

Polymyositis
Endocrine myopathies
Chronic, slowly progressive polymyopathies, (i.e., central core disease, glycogen storage disease)

Episodic Weakness

Familial (hypokalemic) periodic paralysis
Normokalemic or hyperkalemic familial periodic paralysis
Paramyotonia congenita
Acute thyrotoxic myopathy

Exertional Stiffness, Cramps, or Spasms

Leg cramps
Metabolic defects of muscle metabolism
- McArdle's syndrome
- phosphofructokinase deficiency
- carnitine palmitoyl transferase deficiency
- debranching enzyme deficiency
- myoadenylate deaminase

Defects of electron transport
- congenital myotonia, paramyotonia congenita, and myotonic dystrophy
- hypothyroidism with pseudomyotonia
- tetanus
- black widow spider bite

(continued)

Diffuse Muscle Aches or Pain

Postviral myalgias
Polymyalgia rheumatica with or without giant-cell arteritis
Connective tissue diseases (rheumatoid arthritis, systemic lupus erythematosus, polyarteritis nodosa, polymyositis)
Trichinosis
Myopathy of myoglobinuria and McArdle's syndrome
Myopathy with hypoglycemia
Bornholm's disease
Hypophosphatemia
Hypothyroidism
Chronic fatigue syndrome

Elevated Muscle Enzymes Without Overt Weakness

Repeated muscle trauma, i.e., injections
Hypothyroidism
Asymptomatic polymyositis
Malignant neuroleptic syndrome

TABLE 16–2. WEAKNESS, MUSCLE PAIN, AND MUSCLE CRAMPS — RED FLAGS

History	Potential Implication
Constitutional or extramuscular symptoms	Infection, inflammatory muscle disease, paraneoplastic syndrome
Menstrual dysfunction, change in libido, body hair	Endocrinopathy
Medication use	? drug-induced
Abrupt onset	Internal derangement, neurovascular
Severe pain	Neurogenic
Exercise induced	Metabolic
Generalized weakness	Metabolic, primary muscle disorder
Dark, red urine	Rhadomyolysis
Physical Exam	
Stigmata of Cushing's, Addison's, hypothyroidism	Endocrinopathy
Neurovascular deficit	Neurovascular cause

secondary myopathies. Proximal and distal myopathy is seen in inclusion-body myositis. Bulbar weakness involving small muscles of the eye and swallowing are suggestive of myasthenia. When asymmetric bulbar musculature is involved, think about cranial neuropathies and brain-stein lesions. Weakness that is symmetric, distal, and bulbar suggests amyotrophic lateral sclerosis.

The regional distribution of cramps can be diagnostic in the sense that 99% of benign cramps are asymmetric and distal (i.e., the common nocturnal calf cramp or foot cramp). Cramps in funny places (i.e., abdominal cramps or upper arm) in the absence of overuse or unusual use suggests primary or secondary myopathy.

Cramps that are related to the use of specific muscle groups are extremely suggestive of myopathies with specific enzyme deficiency, usually involving the oxidative phosphorylation of ATP. These include McArdle's phosphofructokinase deficiency, carnitine palmitoyl tranferase deficiency, myoadenylate deaminase deficiency, and problems with electron transport in the cytochrome oxidase pathway of muscle metabolism. These, as one might imagine, are exceedingly rare, even in referral practices. However, since some may be treatable by dietary manipulations, the possibility must be kept in mind. A screening exam for induced cramps after ischemic exercise may help in selecting out these patients for further evaluation (see below).

Weakness due to true loss of muscle power should be distinguished from asthenia and from easy fatigability. Weakness comes from the loss of muscle power, but patients who have generalized weakness may interpret this symptom as not feeling well (asthenia), as decreased stamina and endurance, or as fatigability. In a given individual, the history may not be terribly helpful and the issue is best resolved by formal muscle testing. People with primary myopathies of any sort have fatigability of strength. Repetitive use of the muscle groups should induce fatigability. Some muscle disorders are distinguished by an abnormal reaction to repetitive electrical stimulation or repetitive use in which paradoxically the contractions become more intense after repetition. These are the myotonias (congenital myotonia, myotonia dystrophica, and paramyotonia).

In a paraneoplastic neuromuscular condition, the Eaton–Lambert syndrome, repetitive electrical stimulation results in increased contractions, but clinically the repetitive use does not fatigue, as in muscle disorders. Clinical fatigability with repetitive use, or at the end of the day, is most common with myasthenia gravis and amyotrophic lateral sclerosis, and is less apparent with primary muscle disease.

Muscle-strength examination is subjective and the clinician who needs to follow muscle strength accurately should attempt to quantitate muscle strength more finely. Techniques to quantitiate strength include Cybex measurement, a grip-strength meter, or using a weak muscle in a standardized activity to see how many repetitions a patient can do (i.e., number of times one can get up from a chair in 30 seconds). Respiratory muscles might be followed by testing vital capacity.

In asymmetric weakness, the muscle bulk should be assessed. Acutely, diminished strength may not be accompanied by atrophy, but with chronic lesions, particularly those caused by peripheral neuropathies or disuse, noticeable atrophy may be apparent within 3 to 6 weeks of the event.

Tenderness on palpation of muscles is not found frequently in practice and is unusual even in inflammatory myopathies (polymyositis, dermatomyositis). Rather, patients complain of muscle pain and myalgias at rest and with use of the muscles. Muscle tenderness on palpation should make one think of Trichinella infections of the muscle (myonecrosis), rhabdomyolysis, or compartment syndromes.

Fasciculations or muscle twitches during rest combined with muscle weakness and atrophy usually signifies motor neuron disease (amyotrophic lateral

TABLE 16–3. INITIAL LABORATORY EVALUATION OF PATIENTS WITH WEAKNESS OR CRAMPS

Creatine phosphokinase
Aldolase
24-hour urine for creatine
Myoglobin
Thyroid function tests (TSH, T_4)
Sodium, potassium
Calcium, phosphate
Magnesium
Complete blood count, differential
Westergren erythrocyte sedimentation rate

sclerosis, progressive bulbar palsy), but may also be seen in other disorders of the grey matter of the spinal cord, including syringomyelia or tumor, lesions of the anterior horn, ruptured disc, or in peripheral neuropathy. Widespread fasciculations occur after poisoning with pesticides containing organophosphates, severe dehydration (such as after vigorous exercise or running), or overdoses of neostigmine.

In primary care practice, one is more likely to hear complaints of fasciculation or a rippling or twitching sensation of the muscles in which no actual movements are observable and there is no associated weakness, atrophy, or creatine phosphokinase elevation. This is a common benign symptom (without a diagnosis) and needs no evaluation other than a good examination and follow-up. Closely allied is the syndrome of benign fasciculations in which fasciculations may be seen sporadically but without weakness or atrophy. Myokymia is a less common form of benign fasciculation in which there are repeated twitches giving the appearance of rippling muscles; it is diagnosed by electromyopathy.

Nailfold capillary microscopy done with a handheld 30 to 40x illuminated microscope can suggest scleroderma, dermato/polymyositis, or systemic lupus erythematosus. This is described in Chapter 14.

In patients with repeated cramps or muscle pain with exercise, the ischemic exercise test can be helpful. In this screening test, serum lactate (pyruvate) is drawn from the arm after exercising the forearm for 3 minutes with a blood pressure cuff pumped over the systolic presure. This provocative test can identify patients with potential metabolic myopathies and excludes people with myositis and other forms of myopathies. One should refer a patient on for specific identification of the metabolic defect.

LABORATORY EVALUATION (TABLE 16–3)

Incisive laboratory evaluation of patients with muscle weakness or cramps can be done inexpensively and is dictate by the clinical situation. If a patient has a mild nonprogressive weakness and has no constitutional symptoms, an outpatient evaluation in preparation for a referral includes: thyroid function, creatine phosphokinase, aldolase, sodium, potassium, calcium, phosphate, magnesium, complete blood count, differential, and sedimentation rate test.

If a good diagnostic laboratory is available, urinary myoglobin and creatine tests are also useful. The LDH and SGOT tests are nondiagnostic. Newer autoantibodies (PM_1, Jo) thought to be more specific for myositis and conditions associated with myositis exist, but these should be left in the hands of the specialist to order and to interpret. Serological evaluations in connective tissue diseases are poorly standardized in many labs and are never diagnostic in and of themselves. A positive test can be more alarming to the patient than it is useful in diagnosis.

WHEN TO REFER

If the patient has muscle symptoms and is sick, an expeditious referral is indicated. These patients may have systemic illness in which muscle symptoms may only be a trivial part of the clinical picture. The laboratory evaluation is to get at other organs that might be involved but are not obvious on clinical grounds. The battery in Table 15–3 in the chapter on vasculitis should be done.

For patients who have ambiguous symptoms of muscle pain and weakness in which the neurological and muscular components are difficult to separate, an electromyogram done by a skilled examiner guided by specific clinical information can help identify whether the symptoms are due to, for instance, radiculopathy or a primary muscle disorder. It is also a useful test to locate involved muscle for biopsy, which confirms the diagnosis of myositis, but one should be careful not to biopsy the exact site that has been studied by needle electromyography because the inflammation from the needle puncture induces an artifactual infiltrate of mononuclear cells and lymphocytes.

For patients who have focal, asymmetric, fixed, nonprogressive symptoms, there is very little that needs to be done from a diagnostic point of view with the exception of an electromylogram.

Of over 70 disorders that cause weakness, cramps, or muscle aches and pains, few will present in the lifetime of a practitioner with an unselected practice, and most of these will be diagnosed specifically and will be primarily managed by the specialist. The general physician's job is to exclude treatable causes such as drug-or toxin-induced myopathies and myopathy associated with endocrine disorders.

When all is said and done, the most common complaint coming into the office will be nocturnal leg cramps, usually of the gastrocnemius, soleus, or intrinsic muscles of the foot. These are distinguished by the fact that they occur at night, usually involve only one side, and are not provoked by use. Nocturnal leg muscle cramps are due to the sudden contraction of the calf muscle with the foot passively plantar flexed. Therefore, the prevention and treatment of these involves stretching these muscles prior to going to bed and using a foot board to make sure that the ankle is not plantar flexed.

The majority of patients will respond to this simple preventive treatment, but some may also require medication such as quinine sulfate 300 mg twice daily or at bedtime, which seems to work in about 80% of the cases. If cramps are related to recent increased activity or are only sporadic, no further workup or evaluation is necessary. If cramps occur in other extremities or other muscle groups, then a general workup for a myopathy should be started (Table 16–3).

REFERENCES

Adams RD: *Diseases of Muscle*. 3rd edition. Harper & Row, Hagerstown, MD, 1975.

ARA Glossary Committee: *Dictionary of the Rheumatic Diseases: Vol II: Diagnostic Testing*. Contact Associates New York, 1985.

Kagen LJ: Approach to the patient with myopathy. Bull Rheum Dis 33:1–8, 1983.

Index